AF386309

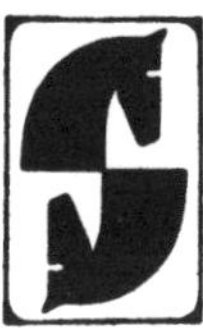

Recent Results in Cancer Research

Fortschritte der Krebsforschung

Progrès dans les recherches sur le cancer

28

Edited by

*V. G. Allfrey, New York · M. Allgöwer, Basel · K. H. Bauer, Heidelberg
I. Berenblum, Rehovoth · F. Bergel, Jersey · J. Bernard, Paris · W. Bernhard, Villejuif · N. N. Blokhin, Moskva · H. E. Bock, Tübingen · P. Bucalossi, Milano · A. V. Chaklin, Moskva · M. Chorazy, Gliwice · G. J. Cunningham, Richmond · W. Dameshek †, Boston · M. Dargent, Lyon · G. Della Porta, Milano · P. Denoix, Villejuif · R. Dulbecco, La Jolla · H. Eagle, New York
R. Eker, Oslo · P. Grabar, Paris · H. Hamperl, Bonn · R. J. C. Harris, London
E. Hecker, Heidelberg · R. Herbeuval, Nancy · J. Higginson, Lyon
W. C. Hueper, Fort Myers · H. Isliker, Lausanne · D. A. Karnofsky †, New York · J. Kieler, København · G. Klein, Stockholm · H. Koprowski, Philadelphia · L. G. Koss, New York · G. Martz, Zürich · G. Mathé, Villejuif
O. Mühlbock, Amsterdam · W. Nakahara, Tokyo · V. R. Potter, Madison
A. B. Sabin, Rehovoth · L. Sachs, Rehovoth · E. A. Saxén, Helsinki
W. Szybalski, Madison · H. Tagnon, Bruxelles · R. M. Taylor, Toronto
A. Tissières, Genève · E. Uehlinger, Zürich · R. W. Wissler, Chicago
T. Yoshida, Tokyo*

Editor in chief

P. Rentchnick, Genève

Springer-Verlag New York · Heidelberg · Berlin 1970

Edward S. Meek

Antitumour and Antiviral Substances of Natural Origin

Springer-Verlag New York · Heidelberg · Berlin 1970

Edward S. Meek, M D, Ch B, MRC Path, Clinical Lecturer in Medical Microbiology, University of Bristol, Honorary Consultant in Virology to the United Bristol Hospitals

Sponsored by the Swiss League against Cancer

ISBN 978-3-642-46238-2   ISBN 978-3-642-46236-8 (eBook)
DOI 10.1007/978-3-642-46236-8

To
Pamela and Patricia

Contents

Acknowledgments

I should like to take this opportunity to express my gratitude to both Hoechst Pharmaceuticals and the British Empire Cancer Campagin for Research for their generous financial support of certain studies in this field. In addition, I wish to thank Miss M. M. M. SMITH and her staff for their help in typing.

1. General Considerations

In the last few years, an increasing number of viruses have been identified which are implicated in the development of tumours. It cannot be assumed that their action in all cases is necessarily direct, and even if it were, then their oncogenic effect may be dependent on, or modified by, other factors such as genetic resistance or hormone levels.

Whilst no human cancer has yet been shown to be caused by a virus, it is difficult to believe that man is an exception to the widespread phenomenon of virus-induction of tumours seen in other mammals, amphibia and birds. Experimentally, human viruses have been shown to be capable of provoking cancers in animals. Also, human cells grown in vitro have been shown to undergo "transformation" after infection by oncogenic viruses.

On this indirect evidence it seems probable that at least some human tumours may be shown to be dependent in some way on a virus infection. From experimental work on animals it is clear that some oncogenic viruses may lie dormant within the body for a period extending over an appreciable part of a lifetime. At a later stage the virus may be activated through exposure of the host cells to certain chemicals or radiation; in many respects the position resembles that of lysogeny in bacteria although there are important differences.

Whilst the behaviour of a virus as an oncogenic agent differs considerably from that of a virus in the common infectious diseases, nevertheless, an antiviral substance effective in treatment of the latter may also prove effective at some stage in the treatment of a virus-induced tumour.

Apart from the question of a common type of aetiological agent, the design of a screening programme for active antiviral agents resembles fairly closely that for anticancer substances. Again, the source material for both in a random screen will be similar. In the case of both cancer (whether induced by virus or not) and straightforward viral infection, there are excellent reasons for seeking agents which selectively inhibit the replication or function of particular types or portions of nucleic acid within cells. POTTER (1964) has discussed comprehensively how the development of cancer cells might be controlled through regulation of gene expression.

No attempt is made here to cover the synthetic drugs formulated for possible activity in the treatment of either cancer or viral diseases; the purpose is to consider only those agents derived from natural sources. It may well be that in due course, some of the naturally occurring drugs may be synthesised or modified and possibly improved on by the introduction of more effective analogues; in another field the extension of the penicillin range of antibiotics is an example of this kind of development.

Intrinsically linked with the search for new antiviral and antitumour agents is the choice of suitable screening systems. For the former this lies plainly between the use of in vivo and in vitro tests. It can be argued that the in vivo tests save considerable time and effort since compounds which fail to produce an effect in these conditions will not be of clinical use; from this point of view, preliminary in vitro study of such agents is wasted effort. On the other hand, in vitro tests are both less expensive and more convenient for the screening of large numbers of test substances. Inevitably, many agents show positive results when tried in vitro, but prove subsequently ineffective or otherwise unsuitable in animal experiments. A substantial wastage rate is to be expected from the use of a preliminary in vitro screen therefore.

To a large extent, these same considerations apply to the testing of anticancer drugs. However, it can be argued that the use of in vitro tests may be very misleading since the behaviour of cells grown in culture over numerous cell generations is likely to be different from that of the original source from which the line was established. In spite of this, there is a fair correlation between the degree of cytotoxicity seen in these conditions and the useful activity against tumours in intact animals.

The use of animal neoplasms is not free from objections, however. There may be little resemblance between the response of an animal and a human tumour arising in the same type of organ, even if of similar histological appearance. Yet this objection can be put forward also when dealing with human tumours of similar histological type—some may respond well to a certain form of treatment and others show little or no response; the difficulties encountered in trying to correlate the histological appearance of breast cancers with the prospects of their response to hormone therapy is a case in point. Such a tumour needs individual assessment according to its particular metabolic pattern. It is not surprising therefore, that in surveying the results of clinical trials with some particular anticancer agent, only a proportion of a certain type of neoplasm may respond, yet a few sensitive tumours may be found amongst a wide variety of cancerous growths. Nevertheless, a drug which is effective against only a small percentage of tumours may yet be the drug of choice in some particular case.

KNOCK (1967) has argued skilfully and convincingly of the need for assessment of response of individual tumours to a range of anticancer agents at the time of operation. There is a two-fold purpose here; first, to ensure the most appropriate choice of drug for suppressing the growth; second, to avoid the use of individually-ineffective yet toxic agents which can do nothing to stem the further development of the particular cancer in question, but which depress the general condition of the patient still further. In some circumstances, it is possible that the drug therapy may also reduce or inactivate an immunological response which may at least have been restricting the growth in its progress (HITCHINGS and ELION, 1963).

Using a system for selection of chemotherapeutic agents against individual tumours, a wider range of such substances can be considered even though many may be active in only a small proportion of cases. In the absence of such method of assessment, the choice of drug will be governed by knowledge of the relative percentage of tumours of that type which respond; the higher the figure then the more likely is that choice. Here the range of drugs considered is likely to be much narrower, and an effective agent for an individual case may thus come to be overlooked.

The situation is not the same as with antibiotics in the treatment of bacterial infection. In the latter it is true that an assumption can be made on statistical evidence leading to the choice of treatment which is likely to be effective in dealing with a particular organism. In some cases, however, the bacteria may be resistant and valuable time lost if a wrong drug is used, hence the use of sensitivity tests for individual infections. Other than the loss of time, which may yet be dangerous, there is no actual positive damage to the patient resulting from wrong choice of antibiotic since these agents are relatively non-toxic. The anticancer drugs are quite different in this respect since the doses used in treatment inevitably cause unpleasant side effects.

Consideration of recent advances in the field of antiviral and anticancer therapy entails then, in addition, a brief review of screening procedures and of techniques for drug selection in clinical cases.

2. The Design of Screening Programmes

In vitro versus in vivo

The problem of testing is a theory one, even more so for antitumour than antiviral agents.

The first choice for both lies between in vitro and in vivo tests. Many agents which are effective against viruses or tumour cells in vitro are of no value in vivo; the wastage rate is high. Rapid inactivation and excessive toxicity are amongst the factors which underlie the failure of so many compounds in this respect. However, some agents which subsequently prove to be of no clinical use, may nevertheless be of academic value in the study of virus-cell interactions and metabolic pathways in vitro. A fuller knowledge of the relationship between interference with specific metabolic pathways and the manifest activity of a drug is likely to be of value in the development of more effective compounds.

In vitro tests have the great advantage of being relatively cheap, simple and appropriate for the rapid screening of large numbers of test substances. Those which show activity are in a minority and can be selected for more elaborate study in intact animals. Whilst the majority of compounds which are active in vivo are also active in vitro, nevertheless some agents would be overlooked if the primary screen is in vitro. There are two possible causes for this. One is that the agent itself is inactive but is metabolised in the body to an active form. The other is that it may act through stimulation of cellular defence mechanisms rather than in a direct manner. The method of DICE et al. (1965) is an ingenious way to avoid the former difficulty; these workers test in vitro for antiviral activity using serum obtained from animals after injection of the drug.

In assessing the value of active antiviral filtrates derived from soil isolates, EHRLICH et al. (1965) use a Virus Rating which is a measure of the extent of inhibition of viral cytopathic effect at levels which are non-toxic or not very toxic for the host cells. A V.R. of 1.0 or more was used as a basis for further testing. Of several thousand samples tested, about 0.1% were active against the four viruses of herpes simplex, parainfluenza-3, measles and poliovirus type 2.

Once activity has been detected it is essential to decide whether a substance is active enough to justify the cost and time of further testing. The best statistical approach to this problem is by the use of sequential procedures, and the subject has been discussed in a concise and masterly manner by ROSENOER (1966) in relation to the testing of potential antitumour drugs. The criteria are selected on a basis which weighs the chance of missing an active agent against that of including one with little or no activity. Experimental tests should be carried out on known active and inactive agents to ensure that the criteria which have been adopted are satisfactory.

Antiviral Screens

While agents of the interferon class are active against a very wide range of viruses, there are some antiviral substances which act only against a small number. For instance, phagicin (CENTIFANTO, 1965) has a more restricted range of activity and is useful against vaccinia and herpes simplex viruses yet not against some RNA viruses. Ideally, a primary screen should include at least one representative of each major group of viruses; primary in vivo screens for viruses are in a minority at present. BAUER (1966) has discussed the question of possible correlation between the size of viruses and necessary concentrations of antiviral substances; the smaller the virus, the higher the concentration of antiviral agent necessary to inhibit replication.

There are several stages in the life cycle of viruses where an antiviral agent may act. In the first place, the virus is in a free state in the extracellular environment. This is followed by attachment to an appropriate cell—the type being dependent on the specificity of receptors on the cell surface and the antigenic structure of the virus. Penetration of the cell membrane succeeds attachment, and is itself followed by uncoating of the viral nucleic acid, and later by synthesis of enzymes. The next stage is synthesis of viral nucleic acid and protein through the action of the new enzymes. Then assembly of the viral components and maturation follow, with release finally of the new virus particles.

Clearly, antiviral agents which act only on the early stages of virus infections, such as attachment or penetration, can only be useful for prophylaxis. Amantadine, a synthetic compound, falls into this class through its action in blocking penetration of the cell membrane by the virus (HOFFMANN et al., 1965).

In many viral diseases the symptoms follow the main peak of viral synthesis, and in these cases there seems to be little real chance of alleviating the situation except by prophylaxis. However, there are two classes of viral infections which are now assuming importance, and which differ greatly from the picture of acute infectious viral disease. One is the group of "slow" viruses, and the other the oncogenic viruses. The extent of their participation in human disease is not known at present.

The virus of kuru has recently been isolated, and from the long course of this illness it seems possible that an effective antiviral agent might arrest it in its progress. Normally regarded as being responsible for an acute febrile illness, it now appears that measles virus is responsible for subacute sclerosing panencephalitis. Again, whilst the cause of a demyelinating disease such as disseminated sclerosis is obscure, it may also be of viral origin.

In regard to cancer, the number of known oncogenic viruses is increasing rapidly, and it is not unlikely that one or more forms of human cancer may subsequently prove to be induced by a virus. In the diseases where the development of lesions and symptoms is spread over a long period, the chance of arresting of suppressing the effects of the virus would appear to be greater than with an abrupt course of symptoms.

The points of the viral replication cycle which call for particular attention are those of enzyme synthesis and synthesis of the nucleic acid and structural proteins. If one considers the uninfected host cell, it is clear that only a small proportion of genes—encoded as sequences of nucleic acid—are actually active at any one time. There must be, therefore, a mechanism which selectively switches genes on or off; a proposal as to how this is done has been put forward by JACOB and MONOD (MONOD et al., 1963). If this can be achieved within the host cell nucleic acid sequences, then it seems possible that some differentiation may be achieved eventually between viral nucleic acid and host cell nucleic acid.

In some experimental virus-induced animal neoplasms at least, the maintenance of the malignant state apparently is not dependent on continued replication of the virus. Nevertheless, there is evidence that part of the viral genome is present and is presumably active. The problem here is the choice of an agent blocking expression of certain viral genes rather than one preventing replication.

In testing for antineoplastic agents, it is to be expected that the use of cells transformed by oncogenic viruses will increase. Apart from these, however, other cell-virus systems may also give useful information (HUEBNER et al., 1962) (TRENTIN et al., 1962).

The activity of a drug may be due to an active metabolite or complex formed in vivo, and therefore liable to be missed with in vitro studies. DICE and colleagues (1965) avoided this difficulty by combining in vivo with in vitro testing; they gave the drug to animals and subsequently took blood samples for assay in vitro. Rats were used rather than mice to obtain adequate volumes of serum. The doses level chosen was LD_{10} since the agent should be selective and not too toxic; in the initial stages four dose levels were given intraperitoneally. If activity was observed the substance was then tested by other routes of administration. As their primary screen, these authors chose herpes simplex, parainfluenza-3, measles and poliovirus using standard methods of assay.

In the testing of large numbers of substances for possible antiviral activity, metabolic inhibition tests are both convenient and rapid though less accurate than plaque reduction tests.

An agar-diffusion technique has been used for in vitro assay with plaque-forming or focus-forming viruses (RADA et al., 1960; HERMANN et al., 1960; SIMINOFF, 1961). After applying an overlay of agar to the infected monolayer, test agents are applied to the surface on discs or in cups. After incubation for a suitable time, the cultures are fixed and stained; plaques are then counted to determine whether there has been any significant inhibition of growth. It is possible also to apply paper chromatography to an agar surface to demonstrate differences in activity by various fractions.

This type of test is simple, rapid and inexpensive, and in the same specimen toxicity directed against the cell can be measured whilst studying the antiviral effect (LINK et al., 1965). By adding neutral red dye to the culture, cell damage is seen as a narrow zone of unstained cells centred around the point of application of the drug, whilst the wide zone of stained plaque-free cells indicates the antiviral effect. Link et al. (1965) used this method for testing against vaccinia, Newcastle Disease, Western Equine encephalitis and Rous sarcoma viruses. This systems also has the advantage that it can be used to demonstrate synergism between two antiviral agents; this is done with two paper strips soaked in the two substances and placed on the agar overlay at right angles. Alternatively, it can be used to show reversal of an antiviral effect by some other agent. From bacteriology, KUCERA and HERRMANN (1966) have successfully adapted the gradient plate technique.

OXFORD and SCHILD (1967) have used organ cultures for the assessment of anti-viral agents for rubella virus; this method may allow closer approach to in-vivo conditions than the conventional monolayer techniques.

With in-vivo trials, quantitation of effect is a matter of some difficulty. LINK et al. (1965) used influenza virus (Al strain) instilled intranasally in mice (in groups of 10 to 30) and observed daily for ten days. The cumulative percentage mortality was shown and plotted into a log probability net against the number of days after infection. JOHNSON (1965) suggest that in-vivo trials should include study on the effect of a drug on contact spread of a disease such as influenza in mice, thus stimulating natural conditions. The subject of development of drug resistance by viruses has been reviewed by SCHNITZER (1966).

Anticancer Screens

Antitumour testing has presented even greater difficulties. The wide screen used by SKIPPER and his colleagues (SKIPPER and SCHMIDT, 1962) is designed to cover as many different types of tumour and aspects of tumour metabolism as possible. Nevertheless the range of clinical variations seen with even a single type of neoplasm raises doubts as to how many test tumours one should use to stand a reasonable chance of picking up a majority of active substances from a pool. It seems inevitable that some antitumour agents, active perhaps against a limited range of neoplasms, must escape both in vitro and in vivo nets.

In 1953, the American Cancer Society sponsored a project for screening for possible anticancer drugs; this screen included animal tumours and viruses, bacterio-phages, fungi, slime moulds, mammalian and avian embryonic cells, and Drosophila. No single tumour type is known to be capable of acting as a single-system screen (GELLHORN and HIRSCHBERG, 1955), neither can a non-tumour system act as the only screen for carcinostatic drugs. Although transplantable neoplasms may differ markedly in their metabolic patterns and responses from their original parent tumour, yet the modified cells may possibly share some particular biochemical feature with a spontaneous cancer of different origin. Whilst spontaneous tumours of even one histological type may differ in behaviour between themselves, and even individual growths change their response (e. g. to hormones) in course of development, yet there may well be many points of overlap in the metabolic patterns presented by various tumours.

HIRSCHBERG (1963) emphasised the difficulty of deciding on a sufficiently comprehensive range of criteria for testing after reviewing reports on the responses of 479 experimental tumour systems to various compounds. SCHEPARTZ et al. (1967) are now using sarcoma 180, adenocarcinoma 755, leukaemia 1210 and KB cells in culture together with some tests carried out on Friend virus leukaemia, Lewis lung carcinoma, human sarcoma H.S.1, Walker 256 (intramuscular), hepatoma 129, Cloudman melanoma (S.91), Murphy-Sturm lymphosarcoma, Dunning leukaemia (ascites) and P-1798 lymphosarcoma.

EAGLE and FOLEY (1958) reported a positive correlation between cytotoxicity in vitro and antitumour activity in vitro. This conclusion was based on a study of

200 substances tested against a number of cell lines, and was supported by the results of SCHEPARTZ et al. (1961) after investigation of a much greater number of compounds. SKIPPER (1964) has discussed the choice of criteria in the design of techniques for measurement of the effect of antineoplastic drugs.

The induction of tumours by viruses offers a convenient means of obtaining malignant growths for use in testing. In the event of viruses being identified as a cause of some human neoplasms, then transformation of human cells in vitro would appear to be of great potential value; that such transformation in vitro can take place in human cells has been demonstrated.

PIENTA, BERNSTEIN and GROUPÉ (1963) have ingeniously combined antiviral and antitumor testing, by checking in the first place for activity against the virus-induced Rous sarcoma tumour in vivo. This short-circuits a great deal of in vitro work; indeed the activity of xerosin can only be detected by an in-vitro test. Similarly, CHIRIGOS (1964) studied the use of leukaemogenic viruses in mice. GLYNN et al. (1963) used Moloney leukaemia virus and showed that leukaemic cells and the virus were differentially sensitive to the drugs used; they concluded that unless both virus and cells were destroyed by a compound, then erradication of leukaemia was impossible. Testing against both viral and tumour systems, JOHNSON (1965) points out that whilst vincristine and vinblastine are both active against neoplasms, the former is effective in vivo against Mengo virus but the latter is completely ineffective.

The disc plate method introduced by MIYAMURA (1965) allowed very rapid assessment—within eight hours—using the degree of inhibition of methylene blue reduction by Ehrlich ascites cells in an agar medium as an index of cytotoxic activity. The value of this approach is shown by the later work of YAMAZAKI et al. (1965) and DI PAOLO and MOORE (1957). The method has been adapted by MIYAMURA and NIWAYAMA (1959) for HeLa cells in agar medium, and again by SCHUURMANS et al. (1960) for S180 cells who allowed for growth of cells during the assay.

In the technique described by SIMINOFF and HURSKY (1960) and GRADY et al. (1960), the cells are grown on glass and the monolayer then overlaid with agar. The test substance is placed on the agar on discs and the extent of toxicity shown by fixation and staining. However, it is necessary to remove the agar after fixation and any dead or injured cells, and ROSENOER (1966) points out that this may lead to difficulty in reading the results.

The cell culture tube dilation broth assay method of EAGLE and FOLEY (1956) has been modified by SMITH et al. (1959 a). A standard amount of a cell suspension of known density is added to culture tubes, with or without the agent under test. After incubation, the final cell density—in terms of protein concentration—is compared in test and control cultures, the activity of the drug being assessed by the degree of inhibition of cell protein synthesis. A minimal difference of sixfold between the test and control is recommended as the dividing line for a potentially useful agent. FOLEY and EPSTEIN (1964) have made a comprehensive survey of the use of cell cultures in screening for antitumour agents.

BHUYAN et al. (1962) used three methods in comparing the activities of various compounds and found no direct relationship between the results obtained by different techniques. The methods were those of RENIS et al. (1962), which is dependent on the removal of damaged cells from a collagen plate, that of EAGLE and FOLEY (1956), and that of MIYAMURA (1956). A further development is that of GOLD (1966) who has measured the differential anaerobic glycolytic rates of elements in a solid piece of tissue without disturbing the architectural mass. The technique is suggested for testing the differential effect of drugs on both the malignant and corresponding normal tissues, and might be extended to procedures other than anaerobic glycolysis.

An alternative method is that of SCHUURMANS et al. (1964) who use Sarcoma 180 and Detroit 6 cells suspended in an agar layer. Paper strips bearing potential antineoplastic agents are placed on the agar for a time, and the the cell preparations are incubated for two days. The effect is assessed by measurement of cellular dehydrogenase activity.

Three types of neoplasms can be used in vivo—spontaneous and induced (generally transplantable) animal tumours, and human cancer cells grown in conditioned animal hosts. The question of methods of drug evaluation has been comprehensively reviewed by ROSENOER (1966) who has discussed the use of various types of tumour for tests in vivo. ROSENOER points out that it is unwise to rely on published data for the growth characteristics of the tumour selected; a careful preliminary study is essential, using the same conditions which will operate during testing. The Therapeutic Index is LD_{50}/MCD; MCD is the Mean Carcinostatic Dose.

Assessment of the effect of a carcinostatic drug in vivo frequently depends on the rate of survival of the animals, but a more sensitive measure is change in weight. Both tumour inhibition and host toxicity tests can be combined in the same experimental animals (ROSENOER, 1966). VOGEL (1961 a, b) compares the degree of inhibition of bone marrow with the degree of inhibition of tumour growth. BROSS and TARNOWSKY (1962) used a "Toxicity Differential Index" based on the differential rates of increase of tumour inhibition and host toxicity. Using this Toxicity Differential Index, MOUNTAIN et al. (1966) tested 14 drugs against 8 rodent tumours; they considered the method had wide applications but pointed out certain limitations.

Another approach is that of SKIPPER et al. (1963) who introduced the idea of a "Specificity Index"; this depends on the difference in weight between control and treated tumour-bearing animals.

HANDLER et al. (1964) studied the reaction to antineoplastic drugs of transplantable tumours which metastasised in a regular manner; sometimes the primary tumour was inhibited yet the secondaries were not suppressed; such a system could be of value in testing agents for use in advanced cases. Similarly, KARRER et al. (1967) suggested the use of the Lewis lung tumour implanted into mice, since metastases occurred regularly whilst primary tumours were still small.

The general position will be improved as variations in metabolism are defined between types of tumour, and between tumour and normal cells. The example of mouse leukaemia cells dependent on an exogenous supply of L-asparagine from neighbouring normal cells spotlights the advantages which could be derived from such knowledge by stimulating a search for a substance with specific chemical properties. In this instance, the activity was found first (in serum) and the precise identification of the substance responsible followed later.

The Cancer Chemotherapy National Service Centre (1964) has introduced a programme for testing antineoplastic drugs for possible use clinically.

The mechanisms underlying drug resistance of tumours has been reviewed by BROCKMAN (1963), HUTCHISON (1963), VENDITTI and GOLDIN (1964) and ELION and HITCHINGS (1965). VENDITTI and GOLDIN (1964) point out that by combining drugs the onset of resistance can be delayed. However, WEBB (1963) emphasised that when two inhibitory agents act on the same metabolic pathway, no greater therapeutic effect is produced by the two than by one only; RUBIN et al. (1964) confirm this.

The subject of development of drug resistance by viruses has been reviewed by SCHNITZER (1966).

The study of methods suitable for assessment of the response of individual tumours to antineoplastic drugs deserves more attention. DICKSON (1966) has introduced a filter-well technique which has the advantage that the interdependence between epithelial and stromal cells is not destroyed in vitro. A simple organ culture technique has also been devised by YARNELL et al. (1964) for study of the effect of various agents on human tumours.

Although antineoplastic drugs should seemingly be tested against neoplastic cells, yet the use of microbial screening systems have proved to be of value. The simplicity of a screen based on the reaction of micro-organisms has considerable appeal. SCHABEL and PITILLO (1961) have reviewed their use.

Foley et al. (1958) obtained most encouraging results; they found that using as few as four selected systems for the testing of 89 compounds 95% of these substances with antineoplastic activity in vivo also inhibited microbial growth. Some two thirds gave false positives which is not of great importance; only 5% gave false negatives.

GAUSE et al. (1959) has developed the use of biochemical mutants of bacteria as a screen based on the similarity to certain metabolic features of oxidation found in tumour cells.

For the assessment of hormones likely to be of value in the treatment of cancer, BECKER et al. (1963) worked with Physarum polycephalum. LEIN et al. (1962) used the ability to induce lysogenic bacteria as a method of detecting potential anticancer agents, and a similar approach was used by ENDO et al. (1963) who tested many antibiotics, antimetabolites and other substances. More recently GELDERMAN et al. (1966) examined the response of lysogenic bacteria to antineoplastic drugs and reported that in each case the combination of drugs suggested by the bacteriological test was more effective in its antitumour action than the use of one drug alone.

3. Microbial Sources

Substances active against both neoplasms and viruses have been isolated from many species of microorganisms. NEUSS et al. (1957) consider that about 0.5% of all cultures of microorganisms screened against solid tumours show some reproducible activity. In spite of this, however, out of many hundreds of cultures showing some degree of antineoplastic effect, comparatively few have reached any advanced stages of testing.

Actinobolin

The site of action of this antibiotic, derived from a Streptomyces culture and known to be active against experimental leukaemias, has been studied by SMITHERS (1966). Its primary action is inhibition of protein synthesis, and suppression of DNA synthesis follows as a secondary effect.

Actinogan and Peptinogan

Actinogan is a high molecular weight substance isolated from a species of Streptomyces (SCHMITZ et al., 1962), which shows activity against some experimental rodent tumours (BRADNER and SUGIURA, 1962). Peptinogan (of molecular weight 15,000) is evidently the active moiety of actinogan (SCHMITZ et al., 1963); it has a better therapeutic index, improved stability and greater solubility.

Actinomycins

The actinomycins form a group of related substances, the first being isolated by WAKSMAN and WOODRUFF (1940) from a species of Streptomyces. Aurantin is a mixture of a number of actinomycins and its properties have been described by PLANELLES et al. (1964).

Actinomycins contain an aminoquinone group giving rise to free radicals which attack the sulphydryl groups of protein and possibly other targets (KNOCK, 1967). The essential biological action of actinomycin is its combination with DNA (REICH, 1963). HASELKORN (1964) found, however, that there is no binding to either polyribonucleotides or molecular hybrids of DNA and RNA. In vitro, the formation of RNA on a DNA-template through RNA polymerase is inhibited (GOLDBERG and RABINOWITZ, 1962; HURWITZ et al., 1962; FRANKLIN, 1963; GOLDBERG, REICH and RABINOWITZ, 1963); however, at the same concentration of actinomycin the activity of RNA-dependent RNA-polymerase is unaffected (HURWITZ et al., 1962). It seems that the main effect of these drugs results from linkage with either guanine-cytosine pairs or of a sequence of guanine-cytosine and adenine-thymine (GELLERT et al., 1965).

GOLDBERG and REICH (1964) have suggested that actinomycin inhibits the RNA polymerase by virtue of positioning in the minor groove of the DNA polymer. Thus RNA formation is prevented by the complexing of actinomycin with DNA-templates (BURCHENAL and KREIS, 1967).

Interference with the synthesis of protein is also recognised. Since mammalian messenger RNA is fairly stable, GARREN et al. (1964) consider that inhibition of the formation of enzyme protein in mammalian cells is probably due, at least on some occasions, to blockage of the translation of RNA rather than with its synthesis. However, whilst both RNA and protein synthesis may be inhibited, the formation of RNA is suppressed at concentrations of actinomycin which give no effect on the production of antibody protein. Interferon formation is inhibited (GIFFORD and HELLER, 1963; WAGNER, 1964; Ho and KONO, 1965), as is also the synthesis of histone in Sarcoma-37 cells (HONIG and RABINOWITZ, 1964).

A useful method for assessing the activity of an actinomycin is based on inhibition of the growth of HeLa cells (REICH et al., 1962). In sensitive lines of HeLa cells in vitro, a specific inhibitory effect can be achieved with concentrations as low as 0.001 µg/ml (JOURNEY and GOLDSTEIN, 1961).

HACKMANN (1952) was the first to report anticancer activity by an actinomycin (D). A number of these agents have been shown to be effective against several experimental animal tumours, differences in effect resulting from the use of different actinomycins. In general, the response of leukaemias and solid tumours is less satisfactory than that of ascites tumours (BURCHENAL et al., 1960). A table summarising the positive results is given by STOCK (1966).

Clinically, actinomycin is of established value. Indeed, on a molar basis, the actinomycins are the most active anticancer drugs available (KNOCK, 1967). It has frequently been used effectively in cases of Wilms' tumour in children (TAN et al., 1959; FARBER, 1960; FERNBACH and MARTYN, 1966) and regression of malignant lymphoma has also been reported. HOSLEY et al. (1962) found it to be useful, when combined with irradiation, in lung cancer, and REEMTSMA et al. (1959) used it in the treatment of breast cancer by regional perfusion. Beneficial effects have also been reported in the treatment of metastatic choriocarcinoma (ROSS et al., 1962), and testicular tumours (LI et al., 1960), in the latter when combined with methotrexate and chlorambucil.

MACKENZIE (1966) studied the use of actinomycin-D in the treatment of 154 patients with metastatic cancer from primaries in the testis. He considered it to be the most effective chemotherapeutic agent when used alone for dealing with secondaries from embryonal carcinoma, teratocarcinoma and choriocarcinoma, but inferior to chlorambucil for metastic seminoma.

Actinomycin has also been tried for effect against osteosarcoma, malignant melanoma, gastric and intestinal carcinoma (KNOCK, 1967).

A combination of actinomycin therapy with irradiation has proved to be of value in the treatment of rhabdomyosarcoma, neuroblastoma and sarcoma botryoides (FARBER, 1959; TAN et al., 1960). Also, actinomycin D has been used to potentiate the effects of radiation therapy in the treatment of Wilms' tumour in children (KNOCK, 1967).

BROCKMAN (1963) reported that tumours do not easily develop resistance to this drug. Actinomycin D has been used by KEIDAN (1966) in the treatment of 31 children with different types of malignancy. Nineteen had Wilms' tumour; many of these also received radiotherapy so that assessment of the effect of the drug was difficult. In the other 12 patients, some showed transient improvement. Toxic effects were frequently observed. This drug may potentiate the action of X-rays but may at the same time increase the risk of radiation nephritis and pneumonitis.

It is given intravenously and tissue necrosis results if it escapes into extravascular tissues. Toxic effects on marrow, liver and kidneys may appear some days after the end of the course and nausea, vomiting, anorexia, stomatitis and diarrhoea may also occur. The dosage is either 15 μg per kilo body weight for 5 days (which may be repeated in 2 to 4 weeks, or 10 μg per kilo for seven injections). Whilst nausea and vomiting can be controlled by chlorpromazine, other toxic effects determine the cessation of treatment.

STOCK (1966) has discussed the variation of toxicity with chemical structure. Actinomycin can suppress an immune response experimentally, but the effect depends not only on the dose but also on the timing in relation to the administration of antigen.

SCHAFFER and GORDON (1966) have studied the inhibition of growth of poliovirus by this agent and find that the degree of inhibition differs according to the strain of the virus.

When tested against influenza virus (PONS, 1967), it is found to be effective if given within the first $1^1/_2$ to $2^1/_2$ hours after infection; it is thought that it may effect the synthesis of viral RNA.

The effects of actinomycin D on the synthesis of RNA by avian myeloblastosis virus and BA1 strain A have been reported by ZISCHKA et al. (1966), who found it active against the virus only in doses which were toxic to the host cells.

Alanosine

This agent has been isolated from a Streptomyces culture (Str. alanosinicus nov. sp.), and shown to have both antiviral and antitumour properties (MURTHY et al., 1966).

A marked antitumour effect was demonstrated using a transplantable fibrosarcoma in hamsters induced by SV-40 virus, although no in vitro action was observed against the virus itself.

In vitro, activity was recorded against enteroviruses, vaccinia, cowpox and sheeppox, and in vivo significant protection was demonstrated in rabbits given neurovaccinia even when treatment was started as late as 24 hours postinfection.

GALE and SCHMIDT (1968) have investigated its mode of action. The synthesis of RNA is disturbed, possibly through the conversion of inosine monophosphate to adenosine monophosphate. Alanosine has been identified as L(—)2-amino-3-nitroso hydroxylamino-propionic acid.

Alpha Sarcin

This polypeptide (MW 16,000), derived from Aspergillus giganteus, is of interest since it contains a hitherto unknown aminoacid "sarcinine" (of undetermined structure) which is also present in two other antitumour peptides obtained from Aspergillus and is associated with the antineoplastic activity. It is effective in inhibiting the growth of several types of mammalian cells in vitro, and of a number of animal tumours in vivo (OLSON and GOERNER, 1965; OLSON et al., 1965).

Anisomycin

Protein synthesis is reversibly inhibited in HeLa cells by this substance (GROLLMAN, 1967) isolated from cultures of Streptomyces. Its chemical structure has been established and it has been shown that its inhibiting action occurs following the formation of aminoacyl transfer ribonucleic acid, but before the release of polypeptides from the polyribosome.

Anthramycin

Anthramycin is the active constituent of Refuin, and is a derivative of a thermophilic actinomycete (TENDLER and KORMAN, 1963; LEIMGRUBER et al., 1965 a, b).

Following trials against mouse tumours in vivo, and human neoplastic cells in vitro, KORMAN and TENDLER (1965) tested it clinically; they reported at that stage some cases of irreversible shock.

KORMAN (1967) considers anthramycin to be less toxic than a number of other neoplastic drugs, and recorded a positive response in about two-thirds of a group of 86 patients with advanced cancer. It may be of some use in breast carcinoma, but seems unsuitable in lung cancer and malignant melanoma. It is given by slow intravenous infusion in doses up to 1 mg per day.

The crystalline methylester form is more stable than the parent substance (ADAMSON et al., 1968). Anthramycin and its methyl ester are effective in suppressing growth of a number of mouse tumours, and also two human tumours grown in rodents; the survival time of mice bearing various forms of leukaemia is increased.

Asparaginase

Since the demonstration by KIDD (1953) that normal guinea pig serum caused regression of transplantable lymphomas of mice, much effort was directed to the study of the component responsible. This has been shown to be the enzyme L-asparaginase (BROOME, 1961, 1963 a, b) and its introduction to the field of cancer therapy is one of considerable promise.

It is now evident that certain types of neoplasms depend on an exogenous supply of the amino acid L-asparagine which is provided by normal neighbouring cells. In the presence of the enzyme for which the amino acid acts as a substrate, the asparagine is broken down to aspartic acid and ammonia so that the tumour cells are deprived of an essential nutrient.

YELLIN and WRISTON (1966) consider that there may possibly be an indirect action of asparaginase through stimulation of RNase activity or limitation of the availability of asparagine for a novel synthetic pathway in the cancer cells. It has been shown that asparaginase causes a rise in RNase in tumours which subsequently regress (MASHBURN and WRISTON, 1965, 1966) but apparently not in resistant tumours; it may be that asparaginase removes an inhibitor of RNase.

A number of experimental tumours respond to treatment with asparaginase (ROBERTS et al., 1966; OLD et al., 1967) even with complete remissions. It appears also that there is good correlation between the behaviour of the tumour cells in vitro and in vivo when exposed to the enzyme, and this is a matter of considerable advantage when considering clinical applications.

DOLOWY et al. (1966) reported that whereas mice bearing *small* 6C3HED tumours showed no toxic effects when given a partially purified preparation of this enzyme, there was a profuse diarrhoea in mice bearing massive tumours. A lack of improvement was noted by them in mice with neoplastic spread to the central nervous system.

EL-ASMAR and GREENBERG (1966) demonstrated the inhibition of growth of three forms of mouse leukaemia in vivo by a preparation of glutaminase-asparaginase derived from a strain of Pseudomonas, and spontaneous lymphosarcoma in dogs has also been treated successfully with asparaginase (OLD et al., 1967).

A differential effect on normal and neoplastic human cells was demonstrated by SCHREK et al. (1967) who compared the response in vitro of lymphocytes from normal subjects with those from cases of chronic lymphocytic leukaemia. It was found that asparaginase is more toxic to the neoplastic cells.

In view of the promising results of animal experiments, a number of human cases have now been treated with asparaginase and the effects have been encouraging for further trials. The enzyme is given by slow infusion. One child treated by DOLOWY et al. (1966) developed severe diarrhoea. HILL et al. (1967) observed a complete remission lasting six weeks in a child with acute leukaemia treated with the E. coli enzyme, whilst OETTGEN et al. (1967) reported consistent remissions in childhood cases of acute lymphoblastic leukaemia. TALLAL and OETTGEN (1968) have found a favourable response in six out of eight patients with acute lymphoblastic leukaemia, remission appearing within 3 weeks after daily doses of 10—500 IU/kg body weight given intravenously.

So far, there is no evidence of cross-resistance between asparaginase and the other chemotherapeutic drugs. The ability to forecast the response in vivo to the enzyme by means of in vitro tests on the malignant cells is an important step towards the goal of selective therapy for individual cases. This is based on a test (OETTGEN et al., 1967) which measures the incorporation of radioactive uridine or valine into newly synthesised RNA or protein respectively; cells which require an exogenous supply of asparagine cannot, in the absence of asparagine, use these precursors so efficiently.

With the introduction of clinical trials, it seems as if the results obtained in man are less favourable than those in mice, although significant remissions have occurred in many patients. A study of this problem has been carried out by RILEY (1968), who demonstrated that the response of leukaemic mice to treatment by L-asparaginase was dramatically improved if concurrent infection by the lactate-dehydrogenase-elevating virus (LDH virus) took place. The clearance rate of asparaginase from blood was reduced by a factor of 5 to 10 in the presence of this virus; it is clear that the effect of LDH-virus in improving the response to treatment by the enzyme is indirect through alteration of a physiological function.

There have been two major problems to be considered in developing this drug. One is the need to find a rich source of supply. A number of sources are known, but some are ineffective in vivo. A useful source (MASHBURN and WRISTON, 1964) is Escherichia coli; as might be expected, the level of production varies from strain to strain. This organism produces two types of asparaginase but only one of these is effective in vivo. MASHBURN et al. (1967) have compared two tests for assessment of activity of samples from different sources; their results show that one may be more suitable than the other for testing certain preparations.

The second problem is that of the immunological response to administration of this protein. It has been shown that the enzyme elicits the formation of antibody in mice (ROBERTS et al., 1966), and presumably may do so in man. Recently, the position has improved considerably. WADE et al. (1968) reported greatly increased yields of the enzyme using Erwinia carotovora. Furthermore, the enzyme obtained from this organism is antigenically distinct from that of E. coli, which may well prove to be of advantage in clinical practice. The situation now is that clinical trials can proceed on a reasonable scale for assessment.

In spite of the limited nature of the clinical trials carried out so far, there is no doubt that asparaginase holds great promise as a new weapon for the treatment of leukaemia and possibly other (solid) types of tumour.

A wide range of toxic effects on liver, kidneys, bloodclotting systems, brain and pancreas have been reported by HASKELL et al. (1969) after a trial in 49 patients. It is not clear at this stage whether these effects are due solely to L-asparaginase or to contaminating glutaminase or endotoxin.

The most interesting feature about this work is that it is based on an absolute difference between normal and malignant cells. Normal cells contain an enzyme, asparagine synthetase which produces the aminoacid from glutamine and aspartic acid, but this enzyme is lacking in certain types of leukaemia cells.

Bacterial Extracts

GROUPÉ and RAUSCHER (1965) demonstrated that xerosin, derived from Achromobacter xerosis, prolongs the latent period of tumour induction by Rous sarcoma virus in chicks and also suppresses the pulmonary lesions of NDV in vitro. Its action is evidently indirect, however, since in vitro it fails to inactivate RSV.

From extracts of Staphylococcus, GRESSER and GROGAN (1965) derived a polysaccharide which showed antiviral activity. This substance is effective (in vitro) against a limited range of viruses—Sindbis, Western equine encephalitis and West Nile; it acts intracellularly and inhibits the growth of virus even if added six hours after infection of the culture.

CARVER and NAFICY (1962) derived a factor from a Corynebacterium which suppressed the activity of Sindbis virus in primary human amnion cell cultures; this antiviral agent was effective in dilutions of $1:512$ in cultures with $100\,\mathrm{TCID}_{50}$ of virus. These investigators considered that interference took place at the stage of viral replication. Although the inhibitory factor was of protein nature, it did not appear to be an interferon. On testing in vitro against echovirus types 9 and 11, coxsackie type B5, poliovirus type 1, adenovirus types 2 and herpes simplex, no antiviral activity was found.

Later, CARVER and NAFICY (1964) studied the effect of substances obtained from two types of Corynebacterium diphtheriae, C. xerosis, Escherichia coli (3 strains) and Salmonella typhimurium against Sindbis virus, echovirus type 2 and 11, and vaccinia. Escherichia coli (strain 0.111) yielded a substance which suppressed the intracellular replication of vaccinia (CARVER and ROSEN, 1964); it was resistant to DNase and RNase, was not destroyed after 3 hours at $37°\,\mathrm{C}$ or 1 hour at $56°\,\mathrm{C}$, but was inactivated at $100°\,\mathrm{C}$ within 5 minutes.

When investigating the ability of bacteriophage to induce the synthesis of interferon, VILCEK and FREER (1966) found that extracts of E. coli strain B showed activity against mammalian viruses. The bacteria were sonically disrupted and filtered through a membrane with pores of 450 mμ diameter. In dilutions up to 1 in 20,000, the preparation was shown to inhibit plaque formation by Sindbis virus grown on primary chick embryo cell cultures, and was also inhibitory to Sindbis virus grown in human embryonic lung cells. There was also some activity against vesicular stomatitis virus and vaccinia in chick embryo cell cultures. It did not seem to exert its effect through the agency of interferon. The inhibitor is evidently a macromolecule, heatstable, resistant to UVL, ether, nucleases, trypsin, chymotrypsin and pepsin. However, its activity is destroyed by pronase.

Other strains of E. coli were tested and showed inhibitory activity, although purified lipopolysaccharide endotoxin from E. coli strain 0.111 : B.4 showed no effect on Sindbis virus. These bacterial extracts appeared to contain more than one inhibitor since there was also some suppression of both vesicular stomatitis virus and vaccinia, but this activity was destroyed by trypsin in contrast to that shown against Sindbis virus. These experiments indicate that this factor acted on the cells rather than directly on the virus particle. The presence of prophage in the bacteria seemed to be excluded, and the authors reported no evidence of induction of interferon formation by the extract in cultures, although this possibility could not be wholly excluded at this stage. Later, VILCEK and NG (1967) reported that extracts of E. coli potentiate the action of interferon, and that the inhibitor—probably a protein—acts only in the presence of interferon; the mechanism of its action is undecided.

CENTIFANTO (1965, 1968), in considering the source of antiviral substances within bacteria, suggested that there may be a connection with bacteriophage infection, and subsequently demonstrated that λ-phage derived from E. coli strain K. 12 contained an agent active against herpes simplex and vaccinia viruses in vitro and in vivo. The substance, named phagicin, appears to be a protein, and its mode of action does not seem to involve the induction of interferon. In chick embryo cells synthesis of vaccinial DNA is inhibited by phagicin in concentrations which do not interfere with synthesis of cellular DNA (MEEK and TAKAHASHI, 1968).

The growth of Semliki Forest virus in chick cells is inhibited by phospholipase-C prepared from Clostridium perfringens (FRIEDMAN and PASTAN, 1968); the virus is not directly inactivated, neither is adsorption or uncoating suppressed but synthesis of viral RNA is decreased.

Injection of a suspension of formalinised Corynebacterium parvum restricts the growth of the transplantable sarcoma J of Betz (HALPERN et al., 1966); the maximal effect is obtained when the injection is given 48 hours before the tumour graft. The bacterial suspension has a potent action on the reticuloendothelial system leading to suppression of growth of the tumour. A similar action followed the use of killed Salmonella typhi.

The development of transplantable mammary carcinoma in mice can also be delayed by the intravenous injection of killed Corynebacterium parvum (WOODRUFF and BOAK, 1966), and a lesser effect has also been obtained on a transplantable mouse sarcoma by the same investigators.

LEMONDE and CLODE-HYDE (1966) examined the effect of injection of Bacille CALMETTE-GUÉRIN into hamsters and mice bearing polyoma-induced tumours. They found the incidence of neoplasia was reduced and survival greatly prolonged. This appeared to result from the stimulation of antibody formation.

NAKAZAWA et al. (1966) extracted a phosphomucolipid from E. coli which inhibited the growth of some experimental tumours.

From Group A β-haemolytic streptococci, OKAMOTO (1968) has obtained a carcinostatic substance which was assayed by its effect on mouse leukaemia, rat hepatomas and testicular tumour in rabbits. As the S-streptolysin content of the extract increased, so the antineoplastic effect diminished. An oncolytic effect from preparations of Proteus mirabilis has been reported by MURATA et al. (1965).

Bleomycin

This is a high molecular weight antibiotic isolated from streptomyces verticillus by UMEGAWA (1966). Its activity is assayed against a strain of Mycobacterium smegmatis, and it is used clinically as the hydrochloride.

Bleomycin inhibits mitosis in HeLa and Ehrlich carcinoma cells in vitro, and, in higher concentrations, blocks the synthesis of DNA. Preliminary reports indicate that it is effective in treating malignant disease of skin, head and neck, and may be administered over long periods. It has been given by intraarterial, intravenous, intramuscular and subcutaneous routes. Side effects include changes in nails and skin, pyrexia and anorexia; the most serious is pulmonary fibrosis which has occurred particularly in older patients. However, no adverse effect on bone marrow has been recorded.

Common human warts have responded to the local application of 2—3 mg of the drug.

Carzinostatin

KUMAGAI (1962) reported that this antibiotic, obtained from a Streptomyces species by SHOJI (1961), is cytotoxic to HeLa cells in vitro and mouse tumour cells in vivo.

Cephalosporin

ACORNLEY et al. (1967) have shown that Cephalosporin P.1 inhibits the growth of rhinovirus type 5 and adenovirus type 3 in vitro. It is a steroid antibiotic derived from Cephalosporium acremonium Brotzu. NISHMI (1966) reports that cephaloridine reduced the adsorption of vaccinia virus to human kidney cells.

Chromomycins

Chromomycin, mithramycin and olivomycin are related to each other chemically (RAO, 1962) but can be separated by appropriate solvents (GAUSE, 1962). Chromomycin was obtained from Streptomyces griseus by TATSUOKA et al., in 1958, mithramycin from a culture of Streptomyces tanashiensis (RAO et al., 1962) and olivomycin from Streptomyces olivoreticulae 16749 (see GAUSE, 1965; MAEVSKII et al., 1963).

Chromomycin A3, also known as Toyomycin, is the most active of a number of closely-related substances of the same origin when assayed against Yoshida sarcoma (TATSUOKA et al., 1958). GAUSE (1965) has discussed its chemical structure. It binds to DNA much as a actinomycin does, and it is said to inhibit the production of RNA in mammalian cells in culture without affecting the synthesis of DNA (WAKISAKA, 1963; GAUSE, 1965). YANO et al. (1963) reported that it suppresses the information of transfer RNA. Its activity against experimental animal tumours and against cells in vitro has been reviewed by STOCK (1966). Its toxic effects differ from those of actinomycin in spite of its reported binding to DNA. Clinically it has proved to be of limited value, although some objective improvement was obtained by KURU (1961) and ISHIHARA (1961), particularly in gynaecological cases.

Olivomycin has proved inhibitory to the growth of several experimental tumours (ROSSOLIMO and LEPESHKINA, 1964), and has been shown to inhibit selectively the synthesis of RNA in the cells of mouse sarcoma 180. Its structure has been studied by BERLIN et al. (1966). KUTCHKAREV (1963), MAYEVSKY et al. (1964) and KAVERZNEVA (1964) reported it to be of some clinical value in trials, and it is said to be less toxic than chromomycin or mithramycin.

As with chromomycin and olivomycin, mithramycin links to DNA. The action of mithramycin seems to depend on inhibition of the synthesis of DNA-dependent RNA (YARBRO et al., 1966); there is no nitrogen in its molecule. RAO et al. (1960) and MERKER et al. (1961) have reported on its effect against animal tumours; the growth of some human neoplastic cells in conditioned animals is also inhibited. KENNEDY et al. (1967) tested its activity in mice bearing gliomata in view of its useful clinical effects on glioblastoma multiforme and reported some response. Clinically, its use is restricted by its severe toxicity.

Mithramycin is unusual in that it is effective in certain clinical situations yet shows a relative lack of activity when tested against the usual experimental tumours. KENNEDY et al. (1967) have studied the distribution of this drug in mice, using its radioactive form, and found the highest concentrations in kidneys and liver; they report that its rate of excretion is rapid. While chromomycin inhibits the synthesis of DNA and RNA equally well, mithramycin shows selective inhibition of RNA synthesis (KERSTEN et al., 1967); this latter finding has been demonstrated also by YARBRO et al. (1966).

Although CURRERI and ANSFELD (1960) reported mithramycin to be of value in Wilms' tumour, choriocarcinoma of male, embryonal-cell carcinoma of testis and cancer of breast, yet it was found to elicit negligible response in a series of 57 patients reported by SPEAR (1963) although the dosage used caused troublesome side effects. Similarly PARKER et al. (1960) were unable to obtain worthwhile clinical effects. In contrast, however, KOFMAN and EISENSTEIN (1963) found it beneficial in the treatment of embryonal genital and anaplastic tumours, also for cerebral metastases. Continuous intravenous infusion is preferred (KOFMAN and EISENSTEIN, 1963; KOFMAN et al., 1964). BROWN and KENNEDY (1965) have used it in the management of cases of testicular malignancy. SEWELL and ELLIS (1966) carried out a trial on 26 patients with advanced cancer, finding a definite remission in four; they suggest that it may be of value in the treatment of neoplasms of breast, uterus or testis. Two out of a series of fourteen patients with embryonal cancer showed complete remission after treatment with mithramycin (KOONS et al., 1966).

As an antiviral agent, mithramycin inhibits the multiplication of both DNA viruses of pseudorabies and murine cytomegalovirus in vitro, but not the RNA viruses of polio and encephalomyocarditis. This inhibition could be reversed provided that the drug was removed early during the multiplication cycle (SMITH et al., 1966).

Clostridia

An unusual approach to the treatment of tumours is that employing the live spores of various clostridia. MÖSE and MÖSE (1964) injected the spores of Clostridium butyricum and other nonpathogenic clostridia intravenously into mice bearing the solid form of the Ehrlich ascites tumour. The results showed extensive lysis of the tumour. The best effects were obtained by the use of strains able to ferment carbohydrate; those which were essentially proteolytic gave inferior results.

Porphyrins which are present in mouse and rat tumours inhibit the growth of clostridia, but this activity of porphyrins can be blocked by heavy metals (GERICKE and ENGELBART, 1964). Following intravenous injection, the spores preferentially localise and germinate in malignant rather than in normal tissues (THIELE et al., 1964 a, b). Extensive or complete lysis has been demonstrated also in hamster tumours (ENGELBART and GERICKE, 1964).

CAREY et al. (1967) have now tested Clostridium buytricum in mice bearing spontaneous adenocarcinoma, and demonstrated increased survival. They also carried out a limited clinical trial on five patients. These were injected with 1×10^{10} spores;

oncolysis took place in three of these but only in their larger tumour masses not the smaller masses. One patient showed transient benefit from this treatment.

Cycloheximide Group

LEACH et al. (1947) obtained cycloheximide (actidione) from Streptomyces griseus, and a number of closely related substances have since been introduced. These are the streptovitacins (FIELD et al., 1959, 1963; SOKOLSKI et al., 1959; DEDERICK et al., 1963), and E.73 produced by Streptomyces albulus (RAO, 1960; RAO and CULLEN, 1960 a). After study of its structure by a number of investigators, cycloheximide has now been synthesised (JOHNSON et al., 1964).

Reviews have been published by WHITE (1959 c), and STOCK (1966); the latter author tabulated the effects of these substances against experimental tumours. The results of EVANS et al. (1959) and SMITH et al. (1960) suggest that cycloheximide is carcinostatic rather than carcinolytic.

This group of agents inhibits the synthesis of protein, and the site of action may be on polyribosomes (COLOMBO et al., 1965).

Acetocycloheximide (E.37) is several hundred times more active than cycloheximide against mouse sarcoma 180, and is effective also against adenocarcinoma 755 and the human tumour cells HS.1 (MARSH et al., 1960; RAO, 1962). The dihydro derivative of E.37 suppresses the growth of spontaneous malignant lymphomas of dogs (McCoy, 1960). Human tumour cells grown in conditioned rats are also inhibited by either cycloheximide or its derivatives (RAO and CULLEN, 1960 a; TELLER, 1961). DELTA et al. (1961) administered streptovitacin A to 8 children intravenously; no therapeutic effect was seen, but the drug proved to be highly toxic.

HAFF (1964) showed that in vitro cycloheximide could inhibit the growth of many viruses—vaccinia, herpes simplex, pseudorabies, mouse hepatitis, coxsackie, polio, influenza, Newcastle disease, Semliki Forest, yellow fever and Rous sarcoma, but only if used at a concentration high enough to inhibit the multiplication of the host cells (rabbit kidney). The effect thus seems to be non-specific, and perhaps results from a generalised inhibition of nucleic acid and protein synthesis.

Viractin was studied by TYRRELL et al. (1966) in cell cultures and in laboratory animals infected with influenza and viruses of the upper respiratory tract, but they were unable to demonstrate any protection against these viruses.

Synthesis of T-antigen in green monkey kidney cells infected with SV40 virus is repressed by cycloheximide at a concentration of 5 µg/ml (GILDEN and CARP, 1966), whilst streptovitacin A suppresses the synthesis of both tumour and virion antigens of SV40 in BS-C-l cells (SABIN, 1966) even if introduced in the late stages of virus infection. Streptovitacin A is also effective against poliovirus type 1 in vitro.

Results obtained by FALKE et al. (1966) on herpes simplex virus showed that actidione hindered penetration of virus but not its adsorption to the cell.

TARRO (1967) tested the effect of streptovitacin A against poliovirus type 1 grown in vitro on BS-C-L cells. Using a concentration of 10 µg/ml, he demonstrated that it was effective in completely suppressing the production of infectious virus when added up to about half an hour before the end of the eclipse period, leaving it in the medium for the remainder of the incubation period. It seems that in these cells it takes

2*

at least 15 to 30 minutes from the time of its addition for the drug to inhibit protein synthesis; after its removal, protein synthesis is not resumed for a number of hours.

During the replication cycle of reoviruses, two kinds of RNA appear in the host cells, a single-strand and a double-strand form. LOH and CROWLEY (1968) have shown that when cycloheximide is added to a HeLa cell culture shortly after infection by reovirus type 2, the production of both types of RNA is inhibited; when added later it specifically inhibits the synthesis of the double-stranded form. Addition of this substance accelerated the appearance of widespread cytopathic effect in the monolayers.

Cyclopin

This substance is a protein extract of Penicillium cyclopin obtained by NAFICY and CARVER (1963).

In vitro it inhibits the cytopathic effect and replication of Group A (Sindbis, Western equine encephalitis and Chikungunya) and Group B (West Nile) arboviruses. It also lowers the mortality rate to a significant degree in mice infected with West Nile virus by intraperitoneal injection, even when added 24 hours after the viral inoculation.

However, its activity against other viruses is at a far lower level. In vitro, there was no suppression of either cytopathic effect or viral replication in cell cultures when the substance was added at the same time as the viruses coxsackie A. 9, B. 5, polio type 1, Echo-11, adenovirus type 2, and herpes simplex. There was a response by all these viruses, except herpes simplex, if cyclopin was added to the culture medium 16 to 24 hours before infection. It seems to act by interfering with replication; there is no inactivation by contact with virus, neither does it prevent attachment, penetration or release.

Cytochalasins

Four of these substances (A, B, C, D) have been isolated from mould filtrates, two from Helminthosporium dermatioideum and two from Metarrhizium anisopliae, by CARTER (1967). Their biological properties are similar although they differ in potency. On mouse L-cells in vitro they cause cessation of cell movement, inhibition of cytoplasmic cleavage giving rise to polykaryons, or nuclear extrusion.

These are powerful cytotoxins; types C and D exert full effect at a concentration of 1 part in 20,000,000. Their possible use in the field of tumour therapy remains to be seen.

Daunorubicin

Daunomycin and rubidomycin appear to be identical, although reported separately until recently; the name daunorubicin has now been applied to this member of the anthracycline group.

Daunomycin was obtained from Streptomyces peucetius by DI MARCO and colleagues who reported its effect against animal tumours (DI MARCO et al., 1964 a, b, c). It consits of a pigmented aglycone in glycoside linkage with an aminosugar. Whilst it interferes with the synthesis of both types of nucleic acid, that of RNA is suppressed to a greater extent than that of DNA (HARTMANN et al., 1964). The template activity of all deoxyribonucleotide polymers involved in RNA synthesis is inhibited to some extent, but it appears to act preferentially against purine nucleotides (WARD, 1965).

Although the early clinical trials of daunomycin by DI MARCO et al. (1964 a, b) indicated only little promise, TAN et al. (1965) showed it to be of value in the treatment of neuroblastomas and leukaemias. TAN et al. (1967) reported that 60% of cases of childhood leukaemia showed brief remissions from a single course of daunomycin; this could be prolonged by maintenance therapy. A transient effect was achieved also in some patients with neuroblastoma, reticulum-cell sarcoma and rhabdomycosarcoma. The toxic effects shown by this drug are alopecia, depression of bone marrow function and ulceration in the mouth; there is a severe local reaction if extravasation occurs.

Rubidomycin was derived from Streptomyces coeruleorubidus. On mouse tumour cells, DUBOST et al. (1963) showed the LD10/ED90 ratio to be 10.

A preliminary report on its use in the treatment of acute lymphoblastic leukaemia was given by JACQUILLAT et al. (1966); after giving 1 mg per kilo body weight daily for five days, four out of ten patients showed complete remissions, and two partial remissions. BERNARD et al. (1967) have reported it to be effective in all forms of acute leukaemia, and in the acute myeloblastic form remissions appear to continue for several months at least. The best method of administration has yet to be decided; in view of its toxic effect on the heart, maintenance therapy is not practicable. Aplasia of bone marrow occurs often, and seems to be more common in patients who have already been treated with other drugs. The maximum dose is 20 mg per kilo body weight, but toxicity is seen at much lower levels.

MATHÉ et al. have used daunorubicin in combination with prednisone and vincristine for the treatment of acute leukaemia. It was found by MALPAS and SCOTT (1968) to be useful in inducing remissions in acute myeloblastic leukaemia, and compared favourably with that obtained by other forms of therapy. In combination with prednisone, HOLTON and VIETTI (1968) reported it to be highly effective in children with advanced refractory leukaemia.

BOIRON et al. (1969) report that a complete remission was obtained in 35 out of 64 patients with acute myelocytic leukaemia using an average total dose of 12 mg per kilo body weight.

Although too toxic for routine systemic administration in the treatment of virus diseases, its action on DNA and DNA-dependent RNA synthesis suggests a possible limited use. COHEN et al. (1969) have reported an inhibitory effect against herpes simplex and vaccinia keratitis in vitro, and suggest that it may be of use in the treatment by local application of keratitis caused by these viruses, particularly if the infecting virus has become resistant to idoxuridine.

Distamycin A

WERNER et al. (1964) produced this substance from Streptomyces distallicus.

It shows antiviral effects both in vivo and in vitro. In vitro, it suppresses the cytopathic effect of adenovirus, vaccinia and herpes simplex; in vivo, it inhibits the production of skin lesions in rabbits by vaccinia and myxoma viruses. It also reduced the severity of herpetic keratoconjunctivitis in rabbits, and of liver necrosis in mice after infection with mouse hepatitis virus. The activity of distamycin A in suppression of vaccinial lesions in the eyes and skin of rabbits has been confirmed by CASAZZA and GHIONE (1965).

When tested for antitumor activity, distamycin A shows some effect against both solid and ascitic neoplasms in rats, but has a poor therapeutic index (Di Marco et al., 1962).

Fumagillin

This antibiotic, yielded by a strain of Aspergillus fumigatus (McCowen et al., 1951), and its alcohol derivatives (Tarbell et al., 1955; Landquist, 1956) have been found to be active against a number of experimental neoplasms (Sugiura et al., 1958; Di Paolo et al., 1959; Merker et al., 1961 b). However, in the treatment of cancer (Di Paolo et al., 1959), results have been disappointing.

In regard to viruses, fumagillin is active against equine encephalitis, influenza and poliomyelitis in vitro (Asheshov et al., 1953), but not in mice in vivo against influenza or poliomyelitis (Hanson and Eble, 1949).

It is distantly related to the Verrucarol group (Neuss et al., 1967).

Gliotoxin

This substance has been found in cultures of Penicillium, Gliocladium, Trichoderma and Aspergillus. Although active against transplantable tumours, it is very toxic for rodents, and is unsuitable as a therapeutic agent. Rightsel et al. (1964) have demonstrated activity in vitro against poliovirus (type 1), also against herpes and human influenza viruses. However, they were unable to show any protection in vivo against poliovirus type 2 (MEF1 strain) or rabies virus. It has also been shown to cause a significant degree of growth inhibition of rhinovirus, echovirus and measles.

The inhibition of replication of poliovirus in the HeLa cells has been studied by Miller et al. (1968) who have shown that it acts at a stage subsequent to adsorption and penetration of virus. Synthesis of viral RNA is the sensitive step, and suppression of protein synthesis follows only as a consequence of the blockade of RNA synthesis. The concentration of gliotoxin which inhibits completely the production of RNA synthesis does not affect the synthesis of cellular RNA.

Glutamine Antagonists

This group includes azaserine, DON, alazopeptin and the duazomycins.

Azaserine (O-diazoacetyl-L-serine) and DON (6-diazo-5-oxo-L-norleucine) were both isolated from filtrates of Streptomyces cultures, the former by Stock et al. (1954) and Ehrlich et al. (1954), the latter by Dion et al. (1956) and Ehrlich et al. (1956).

The chemical and biological properties of azaserine and DON have been reviewed by Duvall (1960), and Emmelot (1965). Azaserine is bound to formylglycineamide ribotide aminotransferase (Herrman et al., 1959); its action is that of competitive inhibition of glutamine (Levenberg et al., 1957). Several points of interference by these drugs in the pathways for synthesis of purines have been described. Both block the enzymic production of the purine skeleton (French et al., 1963).

Stock (1966) tabulated the positive action of these agents against experimental tumours and has listed several which show resistance. The toxic effects of azaserine in mammals are similar to those of DON. The cumulative toxicity of DON is marked. Azaserine has been combined with 6-chloropurine, 6-mercaptopurine,

6-bromopurine, thioguanine, 8-azaguanine in the treatment of experimental animal tumours, and its effect has been enhanced in some neoplasms by each of these drugs.

Azaserine has been tried clinically but has proved, however, to be of little value (DUVALL, 1960).

In some cases an enhanced response is seen when combined with 6-mercaptopurine; although it is of some value in acute childhood leukaemias (SULLIVAN et al., 1962) the toxic effects are troublesome. KARNOFSKY et al. (1964) found DON and azaserine useful for the treatment of trophoblastic tumours; the former can be given orally and can produce long remissions with slowly-growing tumours; however, it is not so satisfactory as either actinomycin-D or methotrexate for fulminating choriocarcinoma.

Azaserine shows very little antiviral activity (EHRLICH et al., 1954; COFFEE et al., 1954; REILLY, 1955).

Alazopeptin derived from a Streptomyces, consists of two molecules of DON joined by an alanine residue (DE VOE et al., 1957); its effect is evidently dependent on its suppression of purine synthesis (BARG et al., 1957). Although inhibitory to some mouse neoplasms, it is not effective against certain rat or hamster tumours (SUGIURA, 1960).

RAO et al. (1960 a) obtained the group of substances known as Duazomycins (Diazomycins) from Streptomyces ambofaciens. There are three types, A, B, and C. Type A is N-acetyl-DON (RAO, 1961); type B is also referred to as azotomycin. A number of experimental tumours respond to these drugs in vivo, and their action seems to be that of DON and azaserine (BROOKMAN and ANDERSON, 1962).

A clinical trial carried out by ANSFELD (1965) with type B did not give very promising results.

Hadacidin

This derivative of Penicillium frequentans Westling (KACZKA et al., 1962), shown to be N-formylhydroxyaminoacetic acid, acts competitively against L-aspartic acid (SHIGEURA and GORDON, 1962 a, b). It has been obtained from a number of Penicillium species (NEUSS et al., 1967).

Although it has an inhibitory effect on the growth of some human malignant cells in culture in eggs (KACZKA et al., 1962; GITTERMAN et al., 1962), yet it was ineffective when tested in a limited clinical trial (ELLISON, 1963).

Mannans

The induction of an interferon-like substance by the use of bacterial mannans has been described by BORICKY et al. (1967). From Candida albicans a mannan was derived which was active in both mice and cell cultures. A galactomannan from Lipomyces Starkeyi showed a lower capacity to induce "interferon" in cell cultures.

Marinamycin

Streptomyces mariensis yielded this compound which is effective in suppressing the growth of a number of experimental tumours in vivo, and which is also effective in the treatment of X-ray induced leukopaenia in rabbits (SOEDA, 1962 a, b).

Minomycin

This antiviral has been shown to be active in dealing with experimental infections by poliovirus (NISHIYAMA and KATAGIRI, 1964).

Miromycin

This substance proved to be strikingly effective in increasing the survival rate of mice infected experimentally with poliovirus (MEF strain), but it was necessary to administer it before the virus infection was established (MIYAZAKI et al., 1963).

Mitomycins

Mitomycins A and B were first obtained by HATA et al. (1965) from Streptomyces caespitesus, and mitomycin C isolated from this organism by MATSUMAE et al. (1957) and WAKAI et al. (1958).

Their structures have been studied by WENN et al. (1962) and TULINSKY (1962), and the biological properties reviewed by WHITE (1959 b). Porfiromycin is the methylderivative of mitomycin C.

The action of mitomycin C has been investigated by SCHWARTZ et al. (1963), BROCKMAN (1963), and IYER and SZYBALSKI (1963). IYER and SZYBALSKI (1963) put forward evidence indicating that mitomycin cross-links complementary strands of DNA. This action is more obvious in DNA with a high content of guanine and cytosine (IYER and SZYBALSKI, 1964; SZYBALSKI and IYER, 1964; PATRICK et al., 1964). In cultures of mammalian cells there is a preferential suppression of DNA synthesis (REICH et al., 1961; REICH et al., 1963; KURODA and FURUYAMA, 1963); this is probably due to failure of synthesis or inhibition of precursors, rather than to a primary depolymerisation of DNA (SCHWARTZ et al., 1963) although depolymerisation of DNA has been reported by GAUSE (1963).

Mitomycin C has three functional groups—aminoquinone, carbamate and aziridine (KNOCK, 1967). WEISSBACH and LISIO (1965) showed that the reduced forms of mitomycin C and porfiromycin were attached to DNA in vitro in the ratio of one mitomycin molecule to every 500 nucleotide residues. LIPSETT and WEISSBACH (1965) found that the guanine residues were alkylated four times as often as other bases. It seems that RNA also is alkylated by reduced porfiromycin (WEISSBACH and LISIO, 1965), and that the drug attaches itself to ribosomes.

Although DNA is the main target, from a study of the effects of mitomycin on malignant human cell lines (a melanoma and an astrocytoma), LERMAN and BENYUMO-VICH (1965) concluded that the drug also interfered with the translation of RNA to protein. In KB cells, LAPIS and BERNARD (1965) found enlargement of nucleoli and other changes resembling those induced by actinomycin-D.

Activity of mitomycin C against a number of experimental animal tumours has been reported by SUGIURA (1961), and results tabulated by STOCK (1966); not all such neoplasms are sensitive. Better results have been obtained in some cases by combining mitomycin treatment with that of other drugs. For example, its activity against sarcoma 180 is improved by combining it with either 5-fluorouracil or 6-thio-guanine (SARTORELLI and BOOTH, 1964).

Cross-resistance between mitomycin C and alkylating agents has been reported several times (Kurita et al., 1959; OBOSHI, 1959; TSUJIGUCHI, 1960; MERKER et al., 1962 a).

Of the mitomycins A, B, and C, type C appears to be the most useful as an anti-neoplastic agent. DUVALL (1963) found porfiromycin to be of little value in suppressing experimental tumours; although its place in cancer therapy is not established it can be tolerated in man and animals at a dose level four times that of mitomycin C (KNOCK, 1967).

Generally speaking, clinical results have not been encouraging. FERGUSON and HUMPHREY (1960) found mitomycin effective in only one out of 21 patients with advanced cancer. BERGSAGEL et al. (1962) found it of no value in the treatment of multiple myeloma. However, KENIS et al. (1964) felt that it might be of particular worth in dealing with cases of head and neck cancer after having obtained some effect with intravascular administration in 11 out of 65 patients. MILLER et al. (1962) reported responses in a number of patients, and MIRO-QUESADA et al. (1961) found it useful in dealing with breast and lung tumours when combined with prednisolone and sometimes Ajulo's filtrate (from a species of Saccharomyces). Some degree of activity has also been reported against cancer of the breast, lung and intestinal tract, also lymphoma, chronic leukaemia, seminoma, choriocarcinoma and various epithelial tumours (EVANS, 1961; KNOCK, 1967).

MANHEIMER and VITAL (1966) studied the use of mitomycin C in 46 patients with far advanced malignancies. About one-third of this series showed objective though transient remissions; however, two achieved remissions lasting 7 and 15 months. Doses of 100 µg per kilo body weight daily or 125 µg per kilo semi-weekly were considered to be effective and fairly non-toxic.

WATNE et al. (1967) used mitomycin C on 24 patients who had already been treated—unsuccessfully—by radiation, surgery and other forms of chemotherapy. The drug was given intravenously at a dosage of 50 µg per kilo body weight for six days and then on alternate days until either a total of 50 mg had been administered or undue toxicity was seen. Seven of these patients showed an objective response; these were patients with lung cancer, pancreatic, renal, ovarian, colonic and hypo-pharyngeal cancer. However, in spite of their responses, there did not seem to be any distinct evidence of increase in survival, and the duration of remission was brief—averaging about 7 weeks.

Mitomycin C is usually given intravenously (KNOCK, 1967); toxic effects, which are often delayed, include anorexia, diarrhoea, dehydration, fever, depression of bone marrow activity and that of lymphoid tissue, damage of gastrointestinal epithelium, liver and kidney. Those of porfiromycin include leukopenia and thrombocytopenia.

Mitomycin can also be considered as an antiviral agent. ODA (1963) reported suppression of the growth of vaccinia, but felt that this might result from inhibition of penetration of the cell by the virions. At levels of 15 to 30 µg/ml, however, the penetration of poliovirus into cells was not interfered with; but at these concentrations the growth of Mengo encephalomyelitis virus was not suppressed (REICH and FRANKLIN, 1961). Whilst mitomycin C inhibits DNA synthesis in cultured (uninfected) rabbit kidney cells, it does not show this effect in these cells after infection with pseudorabies although the yield of virus is reduced (BEN-PORAT et al., 1961).

Mycoplasma

SOMERSON and COOK (1965) found that the growth of Rous sarcoma virus was suppressed in vitro by the presence of Mycoplasma orale in the culture. This inhibitory activity is not, however, a non-specific effect since chick embryo fibroblasts infected with the mycoplasma supported the growth of influenza-B virus (Taiwan strain).

Noformicin

A study of its antiviral effects has been made by TOYOSHIMA et al. (1966) who found it active against both DNA and RNA viruses.

Nogalomycin

This cytotoxic polyhydroxyanthraquinone is derived from Streptomyces nogalater var. nogaltar. Its action resembles that of the actinomycins in its inhibition of DNA-dependent synthesis of RNA through its binding to DNA; it may possibly differ, however, by linking to deoxyadenylate and/or deoxythymidylate residues in DNA (BHUYAN and DIETZ, 1965; GRAY et al., 1966). Its antitumour properties have been described by BHUYAN and DIETZ (1965).

Pactamycin

This is obtained from Streptomyces pactum var pactum. BHUYAN et al. (1961) describe its activity against certain human tumour cells both in vitro and also in vivo when grown in conditioned experimental animals. BHUYAN and JOHNSON (1963) report that its blood level falls rapidly after intravenous administration. This substance has been shown to inhibit the synthesis of protein in KB cells (BHUYAN, 1967).

Penicillium Derivatives

Helenine and Statolon have both been derived from Penicillium cultures; since both are known to manifest their antiviral properties through the induction of interferon, these substances are considered under the heading of "Interferon".

Another antiviral substance has been obtained from cultures of Penicillium cyaneofulvum by COOKE and STEVENSON (1965 a, b). This substance, referred to as AVS, suppresses the influenzas A and B, also Newcastle Disease Virus, in vitro at a concentration of 0.125 mg/ml, but shows no activity against these viruses in ovo (DAVID-WEST et al., 1968 a). It does not stop pock formation by either vaccinia or herpes simplex, but does reduce the size of the vaccinia pocks. It contains protein, carbohydrate, RNA and DNA, but it seems likely that the protein moiety is relatively inactive. So far, its mode of action has not been defined (DAVID-WEST et al., 1968 b).

Phleomycin

This agent was originally isolated from a culture of Streptomyces verticillis (MAEDA et al., 1965), and is a copper-containing antibiotic. When tested against HeLa cells in vitro, phleomycin was shown by KAJIWARA et al. (1966) to prevent cell division and inhibit the synthesis of DNA. Its activity against a number of experimental tumours has been reported by BRADNER and PINDELL (1962). Phleomycin is bound to DNA, and selectively suppresses its synthesis (TANAKA et al., 1963; FALASCHI and KORNBERG, 1964). PIETSCH (1966) found that phleomycin combines directly with DNA in the minor groove of the molecule.

DJORDJEVIC and KIM (1967) studied the action of this drug on HeLa cells, and evaluated its effect by the degree of inhibition of colony formation. Its maximal effect was obtained when exposure of the cells to phleomycin took place in the G2 (post-DNA-synthesis) period. Progression of cells into the phase of DNA synthesis was not halted, and progression into mitosis was only inhibited after a two-hour lag.

Phytoflagellates

The phytoflagellate Pyrmnesium parvum contains a substance which causes lysis of Ehrlich tumour cells. Its action has been studied by DAFNI and CHILO (1966) who reported the effect of variations in pH and temperature.

Propionin

In the course of an extensive survey by CUTTING and his colleagues, RAMANATHAN et al. (1966 a) reported that crude extracts of Propionibacterium freudenreichii show activity against Columbia-SK virus and vaccinia viruses. Its purification has been described by RAMANATHAN et al. (1966 b). Propionin-A is effective against vaccinia only. Purification of the substance active against Columbia-SK suggests that it may be a polypeptide, possibly with a carbohydrate moiety of M.W. 2,000 to 10,000. Further work (RAMANATHAN et al., 1968) shows that this latter substance consists of 2 active components, B and C.

Puromycin

This substance isolated from Streptomyces alboniger (PORTER et al., 1952) has proved to be of great use academically in experiments calling for the inhibition of protein synthesis, but clinically it is of no value in dealing with tumours.

Its chemical structure (WALLER et al., 1953; NATHANS and NEIDLE, 1963), biological properties (BAKER et al., 1955; KARNOFSKY and CLARKSON, 1963; DUBACH, 1964; EMMELOT, 1965) have been described.

It seems that its site of action is the ribosome. Here it is bound covalently to the peptide chain through the aminogroup of its p-methoxyphenylalanine residue (ALLEN and ZAMECNIK, 1962; ARLINGHAUS et al., 1962; ZAMECNIK, 1962; RABINOWITZ and FISHER, 1962); this leads to detachment of incomplete peptide chains from the ribosomal surface.

ALEXANDER and NAGASAWA (1964) reported that the triacetyl and N3-monoacetyl derivatives lacked the toxicity against kidney tissue shown by other puromycin derivatives.

Puromycin suppresses the synthesis of poliovirus RNA probably by blocking the formation of a specific RNA-polymerase; it also inhibits formation of the vaccinia virus-induced enzyme thymidine kinase in L-cells (KIT et al., 1963).

At a concentration of 10 µg/ml, puromycin fails to abolish the synthesis of the T-antigen resulting from SV40 infection of green monkey kidney cells (GILDER and CARP, 1966).

As with cases of malignancy, it is of no clinical value in the treatment of viruses diseases (WECKER, 1965).

Quinomycin

This complex of antiviral agents (A, B and C) is effective in prolonging survival times and preventing paralysis in mice infected with poliovirus (TSUNODA, 1962). All three components (A, B and C) are of equal activity and all contain quinoxaline. The effective dose, given daily, was $^1/_4$ to $^1/_2$ the toxic dose. It proved to be necessary to give the antibiotic before infection.

Rifampicin

This is an antibacterial drug, derived through rifamycin from Streptomyces mediterraneus, and is clinically acceptable as an oral preparation.

Recently it has been shown to have antiviral activity. HELLER et al. (1969) and SUBAK-SHARPE et al. (1969) have both virus in vitro, and the latter group have also shown an effect against an adenovirus.

In Escherichia coli, rifampicin inhibits the action of the DNA-dependent RNA-polymerase and stops transcription (WEHRLI et al., 1968). In mammalian cells it seems that the cellular enzyme is less sensitive than that of the virus particle, so that viral multiplication can be inhibited without damage to the host cell. This drug is several hundred times less active against viruses than against bacteria, and it seems that resistant strains of organisms may appear readily (SUBAK- SHARPE et al., 1969).

Septacidin

This antineoplastic agent, isolated from Streptomyces fimbriatus, shows activity against mammalian tumour cells (adenocarcinoma 755 and L-cells) in vitro and in vivo (DUTCHER et al., 1963; VON SALTZA et al., 1964).

Sparsomycin

Activity against some experimental tumours has been demonstrated with this substance which is derived from Streptomyces sparsogenus (OWEN et al., 1962).

Spiramycin

Spiramycin was isolated from Streptomyces ambifaciens (PINNERT-SINDICO et al., 1955).

BACK et al. (1964) investigated the antitumour activity of this substance and demonstrated it to be effected against some animal neoplasms. When injected directly into malignant melanomas necrosis of tumour tissue followed; some objective improvement was also seen in a case of Kaposi's haemorrhagic sarcoma.

Streptonigrin

This is the product of Streptomyces flocculus (RAO and CULLEN, 1960 a, b). RAO et al. (1964) have determined its structure which resembles that of mitomycin C. It contains an aminoquinone group, as do the actinomycins, and binds to DNA.

MILLER et al. (1967) found that streptonigrin dissociates the formation of adenosine triphosphate from oxygen consumption in human leukaemic leucocytes. It causes a decrease in cellular adenosine triphosphate and in protein synthesis; however, ribosomal protein synthesis is not affected. These authors consider that the action of this drug on cell metabolism results primarily from the catalytic oxidation of reduced diphosphopyridine nucleotide and the resultant peroxide formation.

In both normal and malignant human cells in vitro it shows considerable toxicity (OLESON et al., 1961; COHEN et al., 1963). In experimental animals this toxicity also proves troublesome when the drug is used in carcinostatic doses (REILLY and SUGIURA, 1961; TELLER et al., 1961; HACKENTHAL et al., 1961). Activity against experimental tumours has been reviewed by STOCK (1966).

Streptonigrin has been tried clinically against a wide range of neoplasms, including cancer of pancreas, bile duct, breast and Hodgkin's disease (WILSON et al., 1961; HACKENTHAL et al., 1961; HUMPHREY and BLANK, 1961); a response has been obtained in a number of these. The methyl ester of streptonigrin appears to be of some value also (HUMPHREY and DIETRICH, 1963), particularly with Hodgkin's disease (RIVERS et al., 1966) and leukaemia and lymphoma (RIVERS et al., 1965), (HALL, 1966). After trying several routes of administration in ninety patients, HARRIS et al. (1965) found an encouraging response to oral dosage in cases of malignant lymphoma and mycosis fungoides. However, a trial with cases of lung cancer proved diasppointing (McCRACKEN and Aboody, 1965).

Toxic effects include depression of bone marrow function and disturbances of the gastrointestinal tract. The dosage orally is 0.2 to 0.4 mg daily or 5—7 μg per kilo body weight if given intravenously daily for 6 days.

Its activity against Rauscher-virus murine leukaemia has been studied in vivo by McBRIDE et al. (1966). They found that streptonigrin, its methyl ester and also isopropylidine azastreptonigrin cause considerable reduction in the weight of the spleen and markedly prolong the survival of mice infected with this virus.

Streptothricin

This derivative of Streptomyces species has been studied by STONE et al. (1965), who found that when tested in vivo against the MHV. 3 strain of mouse hepatitis virus, it increased the survival time of a test group when compared with that of the control group.

Its action has also been investigated in vitro against the A-1 human virus ("hepatitis") (O'MALLEY et al.) grown in primary rabbit kidney cells. Given in a dose concentration of 3 μg/ml (or more) 24 hours before the virus inoculation, it prevented development of the cytopathic effect. When tested in vitro against herpes simplex grown in the same cells, and also against polio virus, influenza-2 and parainfluenza-2, no antiviral activity was seen when using concentrations up to 25 μg/ml.

Streptozotocin

This derivative of Streptomyces achromogenes is effective in suppressing the growth of leukaemic cells in mice (RAKATIEN et al., 1963). MURRAY-LYON et al. (1968) treated a case of malignant islet-cell tumour with streptozotocin and recorded symptomatic relief together with a decrease in the size of hepatic secondaries. However, this substance, which has a nitrosamide structure, induces kidney tumours in rats (ARISON and FENDALE, 1967).

Tenuazonic Acid

This is derived from a strain of Aspergillus, and used in the form of the sodium salt. MILLER et al. (1963, 1964) found it active in mice in inhibiting the cytopathic effect of a wide range of both RNA (polio, echo, coxsackie, measles, rhinovirus) and DNA viruses (vaccinia, herpes simplex and herpes B); however, it was not effective against influenza, Friend leukaemia, rabies or polyoma virus.

Tubericidin

SUZUKI and MARUMO (1961) showed that this Streptomyces derivative is 7-deaza-adenoxine. It is effective in suppressing certain experimental tumours (OWEN and SMITH, 1964).

Viral Oncolysis

A number of attempts have been made to develop the use of viruses as oncolytic agents (SOUTHAM, 1960; MOORE, 1960), the essence of the problem being to find a virus capable of destroying the tumour with minimal reaction in the host. Examples of such viruses have been reported by BENNETTE (1960), and by NELSON and TAR-NOWSKY (1960).

The immunological aspects of oncolysis by viruses has been skilfully and comprehensively reviewed by LINDENMANN and KLEIN (1967) in a recent publication in this series, therefore no attempt will be made here to repeat the survey. These authors point out that the search for such viruses can be directed along any of three lines, namely

1) empirical screening of viruses for activity against a number of test tumours

2) adaptation by serial passage of viruses which are not notably oncolytic in the first instance

3) attempted isolation of "passenger" viruses from tumours showing a sharp fall in growth potential at some stage.

CASSEL and GARRETT (1967) have examined vaccinia virus as a possible candidate for this purpose. After 238 passages in mouse brain, the L-strain of the virus finally acquired the ability to multiply in and cause lysis of Ehrlich ascites tumour cells. NEL and LEV strains were also tested and found to become oncolytic at the same time that they became fully adapted to nervous tissue. These authors consider that there is a distinct correlation between the oncolytic properties and neurotropic properties of a virus. This view is reinforced by their experience (CASSELL and GARRETT, 1967 b) with influenza virus (WS strain) which showed high oncolytic activity against these tumour cells at the same time that it became adapted to full neurovirulence.

Earlier, MOORE (1952) had suggested that a common substrate might exist in nervous and neoplastic tissues; this could possibly account for such a correlation. At the same time this raises the question of the danger of involvement of the central nervous system in attempts to use such viruses clinically. SPEIR and SOUTHAM (1960) suggested that this risk might be circumvented by using an avirulent virus to induce an interference reaction in nervous tissue. The question of immunological reaction to an oncolytic virus would remain, however.

An attempt has been made by WEBB et al. (1966) recently to treat 28 cases of leukaemia and other neoplasms with two types of arbovirus (LANGAT and KYASANUR

Forest). None of these were cured but four benefitted to some extent from the treatment. Webb et al. (1966) consider three mechanisms which might account for the effects.

a) direct oncolysis,
b) interference with an oncogenic virus and induction of interferon,
c) enhancement of the antigenicity of cancer cells.

Zakay-Roness and Bernkopf (1964) studied the effect of injections of vaccinia virus (both active and irradiated by ultraviolet light) in rats 11 days after inoculation of Shay leukaemia cells. The development of leukaemia was prevented in some animals, and survival time was increased in others. In vitro, both active and inactive vaccinia virus preparations destroyed the leukaemia cells.

More recently, McGee (1966) injected smallpox vaccine into 65 patients bearing 165 warts. After some local reaction, 164 of these warts vanished without trace, the process being accompanied by lymphocytic infiltration confined to the dermis. Heat-attenuated and UV-inactivated smallpox vaccine was also tried, but no reaction or regression was obtained with either of these preparations. The author points out that interferon production may be concerned in the reaction.

It seems that the immunological response against tumours can be enhanced through the action of viruses without oncolysis. Recent reports of this type are those of Bismanis (1964) and Apfel et al. (1966).

Lindemann and Klein (1967) immunised mice against Ehrlich ascites tumour cells by a single intraperitoneal injection of pretreated tumour cells. The treatment consisted of infection by an oncolytic strain of influenza-A virus followed by homogenisation and lyophilisation. In contrast, no immunity was induced by the injection of non-infected homogenised tumour cells even if these were mixed with the virus after its growth in eggs. These authors suggest that the virus may exert an adjuvant effect on the antigenic stimulus of an alloantigen in the tumour cells, but that even if so, the mechanism of immunity still remains difficult to explain. In the first instance it is necessary for the oncolytic virus to grow in the cells; mere mixing of virus and cell lysate does not increase the antigenic stimulus. However, passive transfer of anti-tumour immunity can be carried out with the post-oncolytic serum which will react with tumour cells which have not been exposed to virus. The possibilities and interpretation of results have been discussed in detail.

Virothricin

This complex has been shown to inhibit the development of several viruses in vitro. Its activity has been tested by Kuchler and Kuchler (1966) against vaccinia, Newcastle Disease virus, pseudorables and influenza A (strain PR. 8).

Vivomycin and Borrelidin

Lumb and colleagues (1965) have isolated two antiviral agents from a Streptomyces species. One of these, vivomycin (Dickinson et al., 1965), was active against encephalomyocarditis (EMC) virus when the virus was given by the intraperitoneal route and the drug by subcutaneous or intraperitoneal injection; oral administration was not effective. A lesser degree of activity was found with influenza as the test virus in vivo; maximal effect was obtained when the antiviral agent was given 24 to 48 hours before infection.

It showed very little effect in vitro, and DICKINSON et al. (1965) considered that its main action was in the stimulation of host defence mechanisms. Enhancement of its antiviral action was demonstrated in vivo, but not in vitro, when small quantities of the other antiviral agent, named borrelidin, were combined with suboptimal amounts of vivomycin. Borrelidin inhibited plaque formation in vitro by the viruses of Newcastle disease, influenza and encephalomyocarditis; no activity was found in vivo against influenza, EMC or ectromelia in mice. The structure of borrelidin has been studied by ANDERTON and RICKARDS (1965) who consider that it is probably an antibiotic of the macrolide group but with some structural features which are unique within this group.

4. Plant Sources

Plants have provided the basis for traditional treatment of all types of disease, and offer an enormous potential source for antineoplastic agents (HARTWELL, 1960).

Vinca Alkaloids

In this field the vinca alkaloids call for particular mention. The parent members of this group were derived from the white-flowered periwinkle—Vinca rosea (NOBLE et al., 1958). Four of the many alkaloids isolated from extracts of this plant have useful antineoplastic effects—vinblastine, vincristine, vinleurosine and vinrosidine. Their biological properties and structures have been discussed at length by GARATTINI and SPROSTON (1966).

These substances have a stathmokinetic effect, and cause arrest of mitosis in metaphase through interference with the spindle, the effect being more marked in malignant than in normal cells. In HeLa cells vincristine appears to block spindle formation or to cause dissolution of spindle tubules (GEORGE et al., 1965). However, their precise mode of action has yet to be defined. Vinca alkaloids may form several active metabolites in vivo which are responsible for the activity of the drug; a survey of this subject has been made ARMSTRONG (1967). RICHARDS et al. (1966) have shown that nucleic acid formation in isolated cell suspensions is interfered with by vinblastine, vinleurosine and—to a lesser extent—vincristine. Both vinblastine and vincristine sulphate restrict the synthesis of transfer RNA; other reactions have also been reported but their significance has yet to be assessed. Vincristine and vinblastine both exert a marked immunosuppressive effect in the rat (AISENBERG and WILKES, 1964); both antibody production and delayed hypersensitivity responses are affected.

Using vinblastine, objective evidence of improvement has been found in cases of choriocarcinoma, seminoma, Hodgkin's disease and other neoplasms of the reticuloendothelial system and also for some cases of leukaemia though not usually those of acute leukaemia of children. HALL (1966) considers that whilst vinblastine has a definite place in the treatment of Hodgkin's disease, the position of vincristine is not clear. Highly encouraging results were obtained by SCOTT and VEIGHT (1966) using vinblastine in the treatment of three cases of Kaposi's sarcoma.

In combination with chlorambucil, vinblastine seems effective in the treatment of Hodgkin's disease and of ovarian carcinoma, particularly where there are pulmonary secondaries (WILLIAMS, 1964; LACHER and DURANT, 1965). BOND et al. (1966) gave

vinblastine sulphate in tablet form to 51 patients; significant responses were obtained
in 6 of these with acute leukaemia, 14 with malignant lymphomas, 5 with malignant
melanoma and two with metastatic carcinoma of the ovary. They concluded that the
drug was therapeutically effective in this form. An oral preparation of vinblastine
was also tried out by WILSON and LOUIS (1967) on 82 patients with Hodgkin's
disease. They used dosage schedules ranging from 0.035 to 0.2 mg per kilo body
weight per diem; the most satisfactory results were obtained at 0.075 and 0.1 mg per
kilo body weight per diem. Remissions were recorded in 31 out of 76 patients (6 of
these cases could not be assessed). The authors decided that oral therapy could be
used effectively; KORST and NIXON (1965), however, used the intravenous route in
an earlier study.

Apart from these results, it seems to have little effect on most other types of
tumour, although there are a few reports of improvement in patients with cancer of
breast, lung, colon, stomach, pancreas, uterus and cervix, melanoma and neoplasms of
the nervous system (KNOCK, 1967). It is usually given intravenously once a week.
Toxic effects occur in marrow and gastrointestinal tract, and there is disturbance of
function of the central and peripheral nervous system. The level of dosage is limited
by the degree of bone marrow depression; lethal effects may result from bacterial
infection following leucopenia.

ARMSTRONG et al. (1967) tested vinglycinate sulphate—a modified form of vinblastine—in 31 patients with malignant disease. A useful response was recorded in
cases of lung cancer, chondrosarcoma, Hodgkin's disease and lymphosarcoma. The
limiting toxic effect was again that of leucopenia. The therapeutic dose of this
compound is about ten times that of vinblastine. No cross-resistance was found
between vinglycinate sulphate and either vinblastine sulphate or vincristine sulphate.

In spite of the close chemical relationship, there seems to be no development of
cross-resistance between vinblastine and vincristine. Vincristine is capable of inducing
remissions in acute leukaemia in children, and is used in conjunction with ametho-
pterin or methotrexate, 6-mercaptopurine and prednisone in the VAMP regine.
Useful effects have also been reported in neuroblastoma, Wilms' tumour, Hodgkin's
disease, lymphosarcoma reticulosarcoma, together with an occasional response in
some other tumours (KNOCK, 1967). The dosage given is restricted by its toxic effects
on the nervous system. Leucopenia is much less common with vincristine than with
vinblastine (FREI, 1964). There is no doubt as to the value of vincristine in dealing
with acute leukaemia in childhood. SAMPEY (1966) has reviewed an extensive series of
published reports.

LASSMAN et al. (1965, 1966) have reported good results with vincristine sulphate
in the treatment of children with intracranial glioma. Its use led to marked and
rapid improvement in most of the cases treated. Good results were obtained also in
six cases of recurrent radio-resistant medulloblastoma, and the drug appears to be
useful in dealing with astrocytoma. With children, it seems that toxic effects are far
less troublesome than in adults.

SULLIVAN et al. (1967) have used vincristine sulphate to replace pre-operative
radiotherapy in the treatment of Wilms' tumour. In all of four inoperable cases they
obtained clearcut regressions. Nephrectomies were performed 12 to 21 days from the
start of the administration of vincristine; the drug was given for a further period
afterwards. Cases of reticulum-cell sarcoma have also responded favourably to vin-

cristine (YOUNT and FINKEL, 1966). Vincristine is generally effective against lymphosarcoma but vinblastine is not. Vincristine is also more effective than vinblastine in
the treatment of acute leukaemia of childhood.

Twenty-one patients with the African form of lymphoma were treated by
BURKITT (1966) with vincristine sulphate; he found the initial response to be at least
as good as with methotrexate or cyclophosphamide. Ten showed early total regression and 7 others a partial regression. These favourable responses were not main-
tained, however.

Generally speaking, these drugs are not of much value in dealing with cases of
cancer of breast, lung or female genital tract (GOLDENBERG, 1964; STILL, 1966;
MYLES, 1966).

Other Agents

At the present time screening programmes are in progress in a number of centres
using plants as the source material. Extension of one such study to tropical plants has
been made by DIJKMAN et al. (1966). These investigators prepared extracts at 15° C,
removed solid material by centrifugation at 3000 rpm for 15 minutes, and assayed
the dissolved solids by refractometry. Extracts were tested for cytotoxicity against
KB cells in vitro and those showing toxicity at 20 µg/ml received further study. From
a total of 177 species, 12 showed significant activity, the highest being that of Abrus
precatorius.

Cucurbitacins have been isolated from various species of Cucurbitaceae; Ecbal-
lium elaterium L has proved to be a useful source. Several of these substances
(elatericin-A, elatericin-B, elaterin and elaterin methyl ether) are known to exert a
moderate degree of activity against experimental mouse tumours (EDERY et al., 1960).
SHOHAT et al. (1965) have shown that the effect can be enhanced by combining their
use with radiotherapy. Low doses of X-rays and of these substances that were
individually ineffective showed a carcinostatic action when given together. This
group of agents causes changes in the cell membrane in vitro at high concentrations
(GALILLY et al., 1962). SHOHAT et al. (1967) compared the effects of elatericin-A in
vitro on human lymphocytes from normal subjects with those from patients with
lymphosarcoma and chronic lymphocytic leukaemia. Blistering of the cell membrane
was seen in the leukaemia cells at a concentration of elatericin-A only one fifth as
great as that needed to produce similar effects in the normal cells. It has been suggested for use in identifying this form of leukaemia.

Colchicine is obtained from the autumn crocus (Colchicum autumnale) and related
species; demecolcin is the N-deacetyl-N-methyl derivative of colchicine. Both are
antimitotic alkaloids which interfere with the spindle proteins. Demecolcin is less
toxic than colchicine, and can be used to deal with chronic granulocytic leukaemia
but is less useful than myleran for this condition. SETÄLÄ (1965) and SETÄLÄ et al.
(1965) reported that normal mouse epidermis responded to colchicine whilst malignant epidermis did not.

LESSNER et al. (1963) found the tartrate form of trimethylcolchicinic acid methyl
ether to be effective in a clinical trial in cases of chronic myeloid leukaemia, but

toxicity was unpredictable. This compound was also tried out in the treatment of this form of leukaemia by STOLINSKY et al. (1967).

Preparations from the plant Aristolochia indica have been used as a traditional remedy for the treatment of cancer. It is now known that its activity is due to aristolochic acid which inhibits the growth of a number of experimental tumours, and of HeLa cells in culture. However, a clinical trial carried out by JACKSON et al. (1964) proved to be disappointing.

Mandrake (Podophyllum peltatum L.) contains several cytostatic substances in its resin podophyllin; podophyllotoxin is the main source of activity. Whilst effective in tests against rodent tumours, it has not proved suitable for clinical use. Two derivatives, namely the ethylhydrazide of podophyllic acid and podophyllotoxin-D-dibenzylidene glucoside, have recently been examined. STÄHELIN and CERLETTI (1964) demonstrated uptake of their radioactive form by human tumours. VAITKEVICIUS and REED (1966) also tested these derivatives but found the toxicity too great for them to be used as the sole form of therapy.

NAKAHARA et al. (1964) obtained a polysaccharide from bamboo which caused regression of Ehrlich carcinoma in mice, and suggested that the effect might be host-mediated rather than due to a direct action.

A considerable degree of cytotoxicity was demonstrated by KUPCHAN et al. (1967) when testing an extract of Marah Oreganus H. against human malignant cells in vivo.

HORVATH et al. (1967) report that the natives of northern Honduras have traditionally used an infusion of the rhizomes of the fern Polypodium leucotomos. These authors have studied the action of a saponine derived from this source when incubated with tissue slices in vitro and found it to have an anabolic effect. The saponine (calagualine) is formed by a ketosteroid and a deoxyhexose, but is apparently not the same as the steroid inhibitors found in Solanaceae. It is said to have beneficial effects in advanced cases of human cancer.

Antitumour activity from ethanolic extracts of the tree fern Cibotium schiedei has been described by CREASEY (1969). When administered to mice bearing either Ehrlich or Sarcoma 180 tumours there was a distinct prolongation of survival time. This fern belongs to the family of Dicksoniaeceae and is native to Mexico; in a parallel study no activity was found in the unrelated ferns Osmunda cinnamomea or Pteridium aquilinum.

Calvacin is a non-diffusable basic mucoprotein derived from the fruiting bodies (sporophores) of the giant puffball mushroom (Calvatia gigantea) (ROLAND et al., 1960). Tested against experimental tumours in mouse, rat and hamster, it was found to be oncostatic in many. Toxicological studies have been carried out by STERNBERG et al. (1963).

In a primary screening survey for anticancer agents in extracts of the fermentation products of basidiomycetes, ESPENSHADE and GRIFFITH (1966) found that about twelve of the samples showed sufficient activity to justify further study. Many of the genera and families showed activity against a number of experimental tumours.

GREGORY et al. (1966) examined more than 7000 cultures for activity against sarcoma 180, mammary adenocarcinoma 755, and leukaemia L-1210. Out of this number, 55 derived from 20 genera showed significant effect against the first two types of neoplasm. The more promising were Irpex flavus, Poria corticola, Hericium erinaceum, Tricholoma panaeolum and Polyporus sp. A purified fraction from Poria showed activity in vivo against a carcinoma and Sarcoma 180 when administered by the subcutaneous or intraperitoneal route but not when given orally. The acute LD_{50} was 2.3 mg per kilo body weight for a 20 g mouse. Further work has shown the purified product (poricin) to be an acidic protein of molecular weight 100,000 containing 18 common amino acids (GREGORY et al., 1968).

Aqueous extracts of seven species of edible mushrooms have been tested for antitumour activity against Sarcoma 180 in Swiss mice by IKEKAWA et al. (1969). A high level of inhibitory activity was obtained with extracts from Lentinus edodes, Flammulina velutipes, Pleurotus ostreatus, Pl. spodoleucus, Pholiota nameko and Tricholoma matsutake; a much smaller effect was found with Auricularia auricula-judae.

VESTER and NIENHAUS (1965) reported that a protein extract made from Viscum album showed activity against normal and malignant cells in cultures.

Cissampelos pareira yields an alkaloid (cissamparein) which is toxic to KB cell cultures (KUPCHAN et al., 1965). In a recent review of natural antineoplastic agents, NEUSS et al. (1967) have listed lampterol from Lampteromyces japonicus (citing KOMATSU et al., 1961) which is said to be the same as illudin-S from Clitocybe illudeus (citing NAKANISHI et al., 1965), and active against experimental tumours.

NEUSS et al. (1967) point out that the agent derived by KUPCHAN et al. (1965) from Acnistus arborescens L. Schlecht and associated species, which is active against some malignant cells in vitro and in vivo, is identical to the substance withaferin-A from Withania somnifera Dun (YARDEN and LAVIE, 1962). SVOBODA et al. (1966) found acronycine (from Achronychia Baueri Schott) to be effective against a wide range of animal tumours.

The antitumour activity of crude preparations of Narcissus bulbs (narciclasine) was reported by FITZGERALD (1958). A recent study of the antimitotic effect of an extract has been published by CERIOTTI (1967); antimitotic substances are found in the bulbs of several varieties of narcissus.

In an extensive screening programme, CUTTING and his colleagues (1965) found that six out of 130 Chinese herbs yielded aqueous extracts which showed activity in vivo against Col-SK virus infection in mice. Twenty-four extracts inhibited the growth of vaccinia in vitro, and one only was active against lymphocytic choriomeningitis virus in vitro. None were useful in suppressing adenovirus. Later, two more plants—Magnolia kobos DC. and Narcissus tazetta L.—were found to be remarkably active against LCM virus in vivo (FURUSAWA and CUTTING, 1966).

TAKENAKA et al. (1961) prepared an extract from Gentiana with anti-tumour activity. Aqueous extracts of the lemon balm plant, Melissa officinalis, suppress the growth of the viruses of Semliki Forest, Newcastle Disease, vaccinia and herpes simplex when grown in fertile eggs and in chick embryo cell cultures (COHEN et al., 1964; KUCERA et al., 1965). The active principle is precipitated by gelatin and may be a tannin. It appears to react with the cell surface as well as neutralising the virus.

A number of antiviral substances have been derived from members of the mint family (Labiatae). KUCERA and HERRMANN (1967) described three groups; one is a tannin from Melissa officinalis which is effective against Newcastle disease virus but not that of influenza; the second (also from Mel. officinalis) suppressed the growth of vaccinia and herpes simplex; the third—from peppermint—contained antiviral fractions similar to those of Melissa, as did a number of other mint plants.

5. Marine Sources

Both antiviral and antitumour agents have been derived from marine sources.

From the sea cucumber (Actinopyza agassizi) NIGRELLI et al. (1960) obtained a substance which they named holothurin-A; this proved to be a steroid glycoside with antineoplastic properties.

SCHMEER (1964) extracted a substance from the common quahog (Mercenaria mercenaria) which was found to be active against sarcoma-180 in Swiss albino mice and Krebs-2 ascites tumour. This agent is present in the clams in a concentration about eight or nine times as high in summer as during the rest of the year.

LI et al. (1965) found a number of antiviral substances in clam, abalone, oyster, squid, conch and sea snail. This team have prepared two kinds of extract from clams (Mercenaria mercenaria), one in water and one in ammonium sulphate. These extracts (paolins) were tested for antiviral activity against herpes simplex and adenovirus. Two strains of herpes were used for assay in rabbit kidney monolayers; both types of extract showed antiviral effect in vitro. However, when the herpesvirus strains were used for experimental infection of rabbit cornea in vivo, the preparations were not effective. Paolin inhibited the growth of adenovirus-12 in cell cultures, and also showed distinct inhibition of tumour formation by this type of virus in hamsters.

Acid extracts of oysters have been reported by PRESCOTT et al. (1964) to be active in vivo against poliovirus. Mice were infected by intracerebral inoculation of virus. The extract was given either orally or by intraperitoneal injection and reduction of death rate was demonstrated. PRESCOTT and CALDES (1967) have reported on the chemical nature of the active substance in clam liver extract.

JUDGE (1966) tested a clam extract against Moloney and Friend viruses in vivo, and found that the mean survival time was increased in the animals with Moloney leukaemia, but that whilst splenomegaly was inhibited in those infected with Friend virus, there was no increase in survival.

LI et al. (1968) have now reported an extract of clam liver to be effective in suppressing the growth of mouse leukaemia -L. 1210. However, the activity is less than that of methotrexate; for this reason, and also because of its toxicity, the authors do not suggest that this preparation would be useful for human leukaemia.

A number of extracts prepared from various species of marine algae have been tested by STARR et al. (1962). Five of these inhibited the maturation of mouse meningo-encephalopneumonitis virus in vitro; the most active were obtained from Lynghya majuscula and Cladophora.

Kelp meal contains a substance which inhibits viral neuraminidase and inhibits multiplication of virus in fertile eggs (KATHAN, 1965). It has protein and carbohydrate components, and may be a non-competitive neuraminidase inhibitor. It may prevent penetration of virus into cells either by direct binding to virus or by inhibition of viral enzyme.

MATOSSIAN and GARABEDIAN (1967) reported that poliovirus type 1 (10^3 TCID$_{50}$ per ml) is inactivated by sea water in six to nine days. Part of this virucidal activity was lost after boiling, and after storage at room temperature. After comparison with artificial sea water, the authors suggest the effect was due partly to chemicals in solution and partly to a heat-labile substance of organic origin.

Takemoto and Liebhaber (1962) have described a polysaccharide present in agar which has antiviral activity. Colon et al. (1965) have also reported the separation of a polysaccharide from agar acting directly on virus and on host cell; the growth of Eastern, Western and Venezuelan equine encephalitis was inhibited in chick fibroblast cultures.

6. Animal and Other Sources

Arthropods

A survey of the possible value of extracts from various arthropods as antineoplastic agents is being carried out by Pettit, Hartwell and Wood (1968). Their source material includes Insecta, Arachnida, Crustacea and Myriapoda; Insecta alone contain about 900,000 species.

The butterfly Melanitis leda determinata Butler yielded an active substance. A 95% ethanol extract of the butterfly (after pre-treatment with petroleum ether and 50% ethanol) led to 65—73% inhibition of Walker 256 carcinoma when used at dose levels of 400—600 mg per kilo body weight given intraperitoneally on the first day of tumour transplant and continued for each of five days.

Similar activity has been found in fractions from Asian butterflies e. g. Catopsilia, Ixias, Pieris, Prioneris and Yoma. In insects, active extracts were obtained from beetles (e. g. Allomyrina dichotomus) and grasshoppers.

Hormones

As naturally-occurring regulators of cell growth, it is not surprising that the effect of hormones on tumours has been the subject of extensive investigations, and hormone therapy has long been acknowledged as a valuable aid in the treatment of cancer.

However, whilst the initial effect on certain cancers may be highly promising, yet long-term suppression of growth may not be possible since the tumour may undergo "progression" (Foulds, 1954) to a hormone-resistant type. Starting from a knowledge of natural substances, many analogues have been synthesised and tested clinically.

Dorfman (1965) has collected and tabulated the results of inhibition by steroids of the growth of experimental tumours.

Wade (1967) has reviewed, extensively and in detail, the chemistry, effects on animal tumours, activity in vitro, and clinical assessment of hormones as anti-tumour agents; it would be inappropriate to attempt to repeat or summarise this work. The substances considered include 17-methyltestosterone, testosterone (and its propinionate), dihydrotestosterone (and its acetate and propionate), dihydromethyltestosterone, fluoxymesterone, 19-nortestosterone, 17-ethynyl-19-nortestosterone, oestradiol, diethylstilboestrol, progesterone, corticosterone, 11-dehydrocorticosterone, deoxycorticosterone, cortisol (and its acetate), cortisone (and its acetate), prednisone, prednisolone, 9a-fluorocortisol, 9a-fluoroprednisolone, dexamethasone, triamcinolone, 9a-fluoro-2a-methylcortisol acetate, fluorometholone, testolactone and ACTH.

In general, androgens and diethylstilboestrol are used in the treatment of breast cancer; Burchenal and Kreis (1967) have discussed the applications of androgen therapy. Both testosterone and testosterone propionate are effective, the latter being very non-toxic to mice; GRISWOLD et al. (1963) find its LD10 to be greater than 1000 mg per kilo per diem. All new drugs of this class are assessed for activity by comparison with the reference compound testosterone propionate. Dihydromethyltestosterone propionate is as effective as testosterone propionate, yet has less virilising side effect (SEGALOFF, 1964).

Diethylstilboestrol and other oestrogens are valuable in the control of prostatic cancer.

Progesterone has been used clinically for the treatment of endometrial carcinoma; VARGA and HENRIKSEN (1965) found that the clinical response was directly related to the extent of tumour differentiation.

For many years corticosteroids have been used in the treatment of acute leukaemia in childhood and in malignant lymphomas. Prednisone and prednisolone are best used in combination with other drugs for the management of acute childhood leukaemia. A trial of dexamethasone showed results similar to those of prednisone. Triamcinolone and fluometholone are also effective. These hormones are oncolytic in malignancies of the reticuloendothelial system generally, except in the case of chronic granulocytic leukaemia. The onset of remission is usually rapid, but the duration is often shorter than with antimetabolites. Given as the sole form of treatment for adult leukaemis, they are not of great value, but are generally used in connection with other anti-neoplastic agents as in the VAMP regime. They are often used with radiotherapy to decrease radiation oedema. HALL (1966) reported that high dosage corticoid therapy is effective in the treatment of Hodgkin's disease.

Published information on the mechanism of action of the steroid hormones has been reviewed by WILLIAMS-ASHMAN (1965). Bearing in mind the theory of JACOB and MONOD (MONOD et al., 1963) on the activation and suppression of genes in the control of protein synthesis, it has been suggested that hormones may play a direct part in the methanism. However, HECHTER and HALKERSTON (1964), reviewing the evidence available, think it unlikely that hormones act directly on genes. The idea that allosteric proteins, which possess two binding sites and undergo a change in structure as the result of binding a metabolite at one site, is worth further consideration. It is suggested that the change affects the steric requirements of the second site, and also the biological properties of the protein. TOMKINS and MAXWELL (1963) have discussed this as a possible means of control of protein synthesis or membrane permeability.

In the case of ACTH, HILF (1965) has reviewed the subject of its mechanism of action in detail.

Tissue Extracts

From time to time reports have appeared of antitumour substances present in various body tissues.

The work of BULLOUGH and LAWRENCE, first reported in 1960, showed that in normal mammalian skin a substance is present which inhibits mitosis. They named this "chalone", and demonstrated that its action depends on its combination with adrenaline and a glucocorticoid hormone. It now appears, from reports from these and other workers, that there are probably many different chalones, each specific for a different cell type, but apparently not species-specific.

Since cancer seemingly involves a disturbance in the mechanism of cell division, BULLOUGH and LAWRENCE (1968 a) decided to investigate epidermal chalone in relation to epidermal carcinoma. Using a rabbit skin tumour, they were able to reduce significantly its mitotic rate with a commercially-produced chalone derived from pig skin. They demonstrated the need to combine it with adrenaline and hydrocortisone, but showed also that some reduction in the rate of cell division occurred when only adrenaline and hydrocortisone were given. Presumably the tumour itself was producing some chalone with which these substances combined. This view was supported by results obtained by treating normal mouse epidermis with tumour extracts; this reduced the number of mitoses to zero. They also observed that there was very little mitotic activity in normal rabbit skin in the presence of a large tumour, and suggested that whilst these tumour cells produced some chalone, their cell membrane was leaky so that they failed to retain the chalone and the intracellular concentration remained low. BULLOUGH and LAWRENCE (1968 b) also reported regression of two types of melanoma by epidermal chalone.

In support of these findings, RYTOMAA and KIVINIEMI (1968) showed that chloroleukaemic cells in rats contained granulolytic chalone but seemingly lost it rapidly. Again, using a commercial preparation of chalone, they showed that the malignant cells were capable of responding by a reduction in mitotic rate.

Meanwhile, MOHR et al. (1968) studied the response of a transplantable mouse melanoma and a transplantable amelanotic melanoma of hamster to repeated chalone injections. The optimal doses were found to be 100—200 mg for mice and 200 mg for hamsters. These neoplasms became necrotic, regressed and finally the area healed.

This field of research holds considerable possibilities but at present progress is restricted by the difficulties of producing chalones in sufficient quantity. The substances described to date are water-soluble, non-dialysable and heat-stable. The epidermal chalone may be a glyco-protein with a molecular weight of about 25,000.

BÜRK (1967) has described a component of normal cells which is of low molecular weight; it has been named anomin. This inhibits the growth of transformed cells in vitro in the presence of a medium with a low content of serum.

A number of inhibitors were prepared by mild tryptic digestion from aorta, tendon and muscle of chickens by PARSHLEY (1965). On testing for effects against 25 primary growths of human tumours in vitro, considerable antitumour activity was demonstrated in a number of cases; these preparations were particularly effective against sarcomas.

STEPHENS (1964) found that albumen and associated material from eggs reduced the growth of certain experimental tumours, and apparently affected the extent of their differentiation.

OTSUKA and TERAYAMA (1966) reported that normal liver contains a substance which inhibits the synthesis of DNA in hepatoma cells, whilst FREED and SOROF (1966) also found inhibition of cell multiplication resulting from the action of a certain type of liver protein.

A carcinostatic agent, which is active in vitro and in vivo has been obtained from liver by NAKAHARA et al. (1963).

Complete regression in about 90% of established mouse mammary tumours was achieved by WATSON (1966) using an extract of calf spleen. The preparation had been passed through a Seitz filter and used undiluted, subcutaneous injections being given twice daily over a period of from two to four months.

A heat-stable substance, insoluble in saline and probably lipid in nature has been extracted from necrotic tissues of mouse sarcoma 180 by MILLER and KINSEY (1967). When mixed with viable mouse tumour cells, the extract inhibited their growth in vivo. The agent remained active after four years' storage at 37° C. A similar substance is said to be present also in incubated normal mouse liver and spleen.

At a chemically more specific level a number of workers have described the inhibitory effects on the growth of human tumour cells by protamine derivatives (O'MEARA and O'HALLORAN, 1963; LUTTON, 1964; HUGHES, 1964).

SZENT-GYÖRGYI and his colleagues have suggested that the rate of cell division depends on the balance between a growth-promoting substance and a growth-inhibiting substance. They propose (SZENT-GYÖRGYI et al., 1962) that these be called promine and retine respectively. Both substances have been isolated from natural sources, including the thymus; they are most readily available, however, in urine (SZENT-GYÖRGYI, 1965). Clams and mushrooms contain retine in relatively high concentrations unbalanced by counteracting promine. It can be used to cause regression of mouse tumours. Retine is thought to be a derivative of the sulphydryl inhibitor, pyruvaldehyde, combined with colloid; it may be methyl glyoxal. OTSUKA and EGYÜD (1967) have demonstrated inhibition of protein synthesis in Sarcoma 180 and Krebs 2 ascites cells by methyl glyoxal.

The results of an extensive investigation by BARDOS and colleagues show the presence of a number of growth-inhibitory substances in animal tissues. About 1140 tissue fractions were tested by BARDOS et al. (1968) against two or more transplantable mouse tumours, together with some 1230 fractions against five microbiological assay systems and a number were examined for cytotoxicity in vitro. Antitumour activity was found in 14 fractions from plasma, red blood cells, bone marrow, prostate, pancreas and thymus. Cytotoxicity was reported from 8 fractions (liver, pineal gland and lung), and a number affected the growth of microorganisms (Lactobacillus leichmannii, L. arabinosus, E. coli). The active substance include proteins, lipids and some small molecular compounds.

GLICK (1967) examined the effect of DNA extracted from various sources on the viability of a number of cell types in vitro. Depression of viability was demonstrated, but the effect was specific and depended on both the source of DNA and the type of cell involved in the reaction.

Nucleic acids, extracted from the lymphocytes of sheep and those of allogenic rats after immunisation against a rat tumour, were found to cause regression of the tumour (ALEXANDER et al., 1967). The preparations contained both DNA and RNA. Regression was usually temporary, but occasionally complete; the mechanism evidently has an immunological basis.

DNA derived from normal thymus was found by GLICK and GOLDBERG (1965) to suppress, to some extent, the growth of leukaemic mouse cells if the two were incubated together before injection of the cells. Similarly, HALPERN et al. (1966) reported that DNA prepared from two rodent tumours when incubated with tumour cell suspensions suppressed their transplantability.

An anticancer effect by RNase has been reported by SARTORELLI (1964).

Since WOOD (1958) showed that the formation of a metastasis depends on the embolic cells being embedded in microthrombus and that without this they are unable to survive and penetrate the capillary walls, several studies have been made of the antineoplastic effects of substances which prevent thrombus formation. These include heparin, dicoumarol and fibrinolysin, and it has been shown that these reduce the incidence of metastases. PACK and colleagues (PACK, 1964) use either heparin or dicoumarol as a prophylactic measure during surgery of cancer. KNOCK (1967) states that heparin has a definite antitumour effect and LARSEN et al. (1964) have described the use of fibrinolysin in advanced cases of malignancy.

Growth of a transplantable mouse mammary tumour has been inhibited by fractions of histone rich in lysine, and also by polylysine (SHAH and REILLY, 1967). However, other histone fractions, spermine, spermidine, protamine and puromycin had no such effects. These investigations suggest that suppression of tumour growth resulted from inhibition of the synthesis of DNA-dependent RNA.

As an antiviral agent, BALANDIN et al. (1966) showed that histone extracted from calf thymus inhibits the growth of vaccinia at a concentration of 100 µg/ml. Its action is possibly due to formation of a complex with the viral DNA.

In vivo, heparin has been found effective by LEHEL and HADHAZY (1966) in counteracting the effect of herpes simplex infection in rabbit skin if given either one or eighteen hours beforehand. The antiviral activity was observed when several different virus strains were used. However, no action was observed against a neurovirulent strain, and the authors discuss a possible correlation between heparin sensitivity and neurovirulence. An inhibitory effect of heparin on some strains of Rous sarcoma virus has been reported by SOLOMON et al. (1966).

Deoxyribonuclease (DNase) has been shown to suppress the growth of a number of DNA viruses—vaccinia, herpes and adenovirus—during their intracellular replication cycle, and RNase shown to have a similar effect on influenza and polioviruses (SALGANIK et al., 1967). These investigators have reported that DNase is also effective in the treatment of herpetic keratitis, adenoviral keratitis, herpes zoster, and has a protective action against the spontaneous development of lymphatic leukaemia in mice if given in the preleukaemic period. They also report a positive response to DNase in human lymphoid leukaemia.

LI et al. (1963) reported an antiviral substance to be present in aqueous extracts of calf thymus. The lyophilised preparation inhibited poliovirus and coxsackievirus in vitro. In vivo, a single intraperitoneal injection given five hours before infection protected mice from the paralytic effect of poliovirus and from the lethal effect of coxsackievirus.

An antiviral factor, active against mouse hepatitis virus but not against Newcastle disease virus, has been extracted from the mucosa of the first part of the small gut of adult mice by PIAZZA et al. (1967). This factor is present also in gnotobiotic mice.

Several mucoprotein inhibitors have been found in blood, urine, saliva and sputum which are active against myxoviruses through their formation of complexes with the virions.

Vaccines

It is well established that both chemically-induced and virus-induced tumours bear antigens which differ from those of the corresponding normal cells. On this basis a number of attempts have been made to suppress neoplasms by immunological means. Two types of response are to be considered—cellular and humoral. Resistance to tumours is mediated mainly by sensitised lymphocytes; serum antibody is an uncertain factor. In some conditions, antibodies enhance the growth of malignant cells rather than suppressing it; this effect probably stems from the coating of the tumour cells with antibody which in turn inhibits attack upon them by sensitised lymphocytes. In this way the antibodies protect the tumour cells which can thus proliferate without hindrance.

Aoki et al. (1966) have reported that antibody to the Gross leukaemic antigen can often be demonstrated in mice and suggest that it may play an important part in the resistance of some mice to the oncogenic effect of the naturally-transmitted virus. Pilch and Riggins (1966) studied the development of antibodies in mice to both spontaneous and methylcholanthrene-induced tumours and reported that antibodies did not appear until after the primary tumours had been removed surgically.

Lindenmann and Klein (1967) comment on the repeated inability to use mechanically disrupted tumour cells as antigen for the induction of immunity. Cells treated by chemicals or irradiation can be used successfully, however, and the use of viruses to enhance the immunological response to tumour cells is discussed elsewhere.

After killing Sarcoma 180 and Ehrlich carcinoma cells with ultraviolet light, Litman et al. (1968) injected the cells into Swiss mice, and subsequently challenged them with live cells. The results showed that a high level of immunity could be induced by three weekly injections of killed homologous cells. The intraperitoneal route proved to be superior to the subcutaneous in the induction of immunity; a significant degree of resistance could be demonstrated after eight months. Mice immunised with irradiated Sarcoma 180 cells were cross immune to the Ehrlich carcinoma cells.

Larson et al. (1966) have pointed out that immunological control of virus-induced tumours might be established in three ways. One is by inducing resistance to the initial viral infection; the second by immunisation against the homologous tumour-specific antigen prior to the appearance of the neoplasm; the third by immunisation against secondary growth using autochthonous tumour vaccine. Considering the first possibility to be the most promising, these authors injected adult female hamsters with live SV40 virus some time before mating. The progeny proved to be resistant to tumorigenesis by this virus after inoculation in the neonatal period. Their immunity appeared to be due to the passive acquisition of maternal antibody which prevented infection. There was no evidence of infection of the foetus from the mother, and no complement-fixing antibody against the T-antigen in either parent or progeny. The development of this type of prophylaxis against tumours is obviously dependent on the identification of oncogenic viruses and selection of vaccine strains.

In summary, it seems that the deliberate stimulation of serum antibodies against tumour antigens carries too great a risk of enhancement of neoplastic growth. On the other hand, the use of injections of foreign sensitized lymphocytes entails the possibility of a graft-versus-host reaction in the presence to an impaired host response. The successful use by Alexander et al. (1967) of nucleic acid extracted from sensitized lymphoid cells as a means of transfer of passive resistance is therefore of considerable interest and promise.

The study of antiviral vaccines is a subject in itself, and cannot be dealt with in detail here. Whilst the use of vaccines is well established in the management of some virus diseases such as smallpox, poliomyelitis, yellow fever, in others the development and use of vaccines is still in progress. The latter group includes rubella, mumps, adenovirus, influenza, parainfluenza, arboviruses; herpes (B-virus) and rabies. In the arbovirus group vaccines are now available against Russian spring-summer encephalitis and Japanese B encephalitis, whilst those directed against Venezuelan equine encephalitis and dengue are being studied. Measles vaccine has now reached the satisfactory position of passing into widespread use, and mumps and rubella may do so shortly.

GARD (1966) has prepared a useful summary of this subject as discussed at a conference organised by the Pan American Health Organisation and World Health Organisation held in Washington, D. C. in November 1966.

There seems to be little prospect of protection in the near future against respiratory syncytial virus, rhinovirus, varicella-zoster, cytomegalovirus or hepatitis viruses.

Interferon

ISAACS and LINDEMANN (1957) gave the name "interferon" to a substance produced by the cells of chick chorioallantiic membrane after these had been exposed to heat-inactivated influenza virus. This substance was found to interfere with the growth of influenza virus, but later it was realised it could also inhibit the growth of other viruses. Moreover, it has since been shown that interferon can be induced by many different viruses, though some are more effective than others in this respect.

Interferon is the name now given to a group of closely-related substances produced by cells in response to viral infections. This family of antiviral agents shows a broad spectrum of activity; however, their usefulness in clinical practice is limited by the fact that interferon must be present either shortly before or after the time of infection by a virus if it is to be effective. Therefore it must be regarded more in the nature of a prophylatic rather than a therapeutic agent.

It is impossible in a work of this nature to consider all of the vast number of publications on interferons which have now appeared. The subject has been admirably reviewed by BARON and LEVY (1966) and by many authors in a book edited by FINTER (1966). Current work has been presented in the proceedings of a Ciba symposium dedicated to ALICK ISAACS (WOLSTENHOLME and O'CONNOR, 1968).

LOCKHART (1966) has suggested criteria which may be applied when deciding whether a new antiviral substance should be classed as an interferon or not. These are:

a) It must be a protein formed by the cell after treatment with an inducing agent.

b) Its effect in inhibiting the growth of viruses must not be due simply to a non-specific effect on the host cells.

c) Its antiviral action must take place within cells through a process dependent on the synthesis of both RNA and protein.

d) It must be active against a number of unrelated viruses.

The property of species specificity was first reported by TYRRELL (1959). LOCKHART (1966) feels that whilst restriction of activity through species specificity is highly suggestive of an interferon, it should not be regarded as essential. The interspecies barrier does not seem to be quite complete as there is evidence of activity in some cells treated with heterologous interferon (BUCKNALL, 1967). DESMYTER et al. (1968) reported that an interferon of human origin was far more active against vesicular stomatitis virus in rabbit cells than in human cells.

The earlier literature contains a number of examples of production of what may be an interferon, but lacking further evidence it is not possible to identify some of these substances. The interferons are proteins, with molecular weights ranging from 18,000 to about 100,000 (BARON and LEVY, 1966), or higher. They are remarkably resistant to changes in pH within the range from 2 to 10. In regard to heat stability, this may vary between the different interferons according to their source; many are stable for months at 4° C. The interferon described by ISAACS and LINDENMANN (1957) resisted 60° C for one hour; the molecule could not be precipitated by centrifugation at 100,000 g but it was able to pass through a dialysis membrane of Visking cellophane. Purified interferon is readily inactivated by UVL (LAMPSON et al., 1963). Its isoelectric point (IEP) is reported by FANTES (1966) as being between pH 6.5 and 7.5.

A number of methods have been used for the purification of interferon. Much of the earlier work was carried out with relatively crude preparations, and in some cases experimental work needs to be repeated with purified samples. The methods used have been reviewed by FANTES (1966). Considerable gains in purification have now been recorded; 10,000-fold for allantoic fluid interferon (FANTES, 1965) and for mouse interferon 6,000-fold (MERIGAN et al., 1965).

The subject of production has been reviewed by Ho (1966). A wide range of mammalian and avian cells have been shown to produce interferon after viral infection. These include those of whole embryo, fibroblasts, cells of kidney, amnion, liver, lung, brain, leucocytes, liver and spleen and lymph nodes, together with a number of cell lines, although some of these latter are poor producers. Diploid mammalian cell lines have also been used successfully. The bulk production of interferon of M.W. 160,000 in human amnion membranes is described by CHANY et al. (1968).

Most, if not all, viruses appear to be able to induce interferon formation, although their efficiency may vary. These include DNA viruses such as vaccinia (NAGANO and KOJIMA, 1958), adenovirus (KHOOBYARIAN and FISCHINGER, 1965), herpes simplex (FRUITSTONE et al., 1964) and polyoma (BARSKI and CORNEFERT, 1962), and also RNA viruses such as dengue (SATHER and HAMMON, 1963), HALSTEAD et al., 1964) and polio (Ho and ENDERS, 1959 a), (ISAACS, 1963). It is seen that oncogenic viruses are also capable of inducing interferon. It is of interest that VAN ROSSUM and DE SOMER (1966) produced interferon in rats by injection of tobacco mosaic and T2 phage amongst other viruses.

Strains of a given virus may differ in their individual ability to induce the synthesis of interferon. This has been demonstrated by AURELIAN and ROIZMAN (1965) using two strains of herpes virus, by LOCKHART (1963) with two strains of Western equine encephalitis virus and by Ho (1962) with two influenza viruses (strains of PRS and WS).

It is evidently not necessary in all cases for the virus to replicate since both active and inactivated viruses have been shown to be capable of acting as interferon inducers. As ISAACS and LINDENMANN (1957) demonstrated, heat-inactivated influenza virus is effective as an inducer. In the case of arborivuses, infection by Chikungunya virus in both active and inactive form (HELLER, 1963) has led to the synthesis of interferon. Ho (1964 a) has pointed out that differences in the method of inactivation may have a very important influence on the results, and some viruses in the infective state may even inhibit the formation of interferon (Ho, 1966).

Whilst replication is not essential for induction, it often proceeds at a low level with infectious virus, or may be incomplete. PAUCKER et al. (1962) has shown this with Newcastle disease virus in mouse L-strain cells and ROTEM et al. (1964) obtained similar results with this virus in hamster embryo cells.

The yield of interferon may vary not only according to the type of virus, but also with the type of host cell. A given virus may induce a low amount of interferon in one cell system and a high amount in another. The ability to synthesize interferon is embodied in the host-cell DNA.

Apart from reports of work based on the use of viruses for induction, there are a number indicating that other agents may also be effective. ISAACS (1961) suggested that induction might result from the action of viral nucleic acid and later papers support this idea. JENSEN et al. (1963) found that both DNA and RNA from various sources provoked the formation of an interferon-like viral inhibitor in chick cells, although it is not clear whether this is actually an interferon. Similar results were obtained by ROTEM et al. (1963) using mouse RNA on chick cells, whilst TAKANO et al. (1965) induced an interferon-like substance in mice after injection in vivo of RNA from yeast and bacteria, and of DNA from calf thymus.

Interferon production can also be stimulated by bacteria. Ho (1964 b) obtained an interferon from rabbits after injection of heat-killed Escherichia coli strain 0.113. HAHON and KOZIKOWSKI (1968) demonstrated a yield from cell cultures exposed to Coxiella burneti. FINKELSTEIN (1961) found that E. coli endotoxin with or without the whole bacterial cell produced an antiviral substance against Newcastle disease virus in embryonated eggs. There a number of other reports (e. g., HOOK and WAGNER, 1959; HORSFALL and McCARTY, 1947) on the use of bacteria in the production of agents active against various viruses but it is not clear in some cases whether these inhibitors are of the interferon class or not.

OH (1966) reported the appearance of an interferon-like viral inhibitor in the body fluids of rabbits starting one hour after the injection of 200 mg typhoid endotoxin; the output was falling by six hours.

The mechanism by which endotoxin induces interferon activity appears to be quite different from that by which viruses do so; the action of virus leads to the synthesis of new protein, resulting in the appearance of interferon activity, and this type of induction can be inhibited by actinomycin and puromycin which interfere with the synthesis of protein. In contrast, the production of interferon-based resistance by endotoxin is not affected by either puromycin or actinomycin (KE et al., 1966), (HO, POSTIC and KE, 1968), and the endotoxin appears to release preformed interferon. It seems that the method of induction of interferon by bacterial endotoxins may differ, however, according to the type of bacterium (STINEBRING and YOUNGNER, 1964). Serratia marcescens and Salmonella typhimurium may release preformed material whilst Brucella abortus may act like a virus. The results of YOUNGNER et al. (1965) show that the action of Brucella can be inhibited by suppression of protein synthesis.

Statolon and helenine, which are discussed elsewhere, exert their effect through the induction of interferon. WHEELOCK (1965) has reported that exposure of cells to phytohaemagglutinin leads to the formation of a viral inhibitor with properties resembling those of interferon.

It has been shown by DE SOMER and COCITO (1968) that interferon blocks the replication of virus early in the circle. The earlier idea that interferon acts by uncoupling oxidative phosphorylation now appears to have been abandoned (BARON and LEVY, 1966); neither does it seem to disturb the cell growth or division, nor does it inhibit the synthesis of nucleic acid. It now seems probable that interferon acts in an indirect manner by inducing the synthesis of another ("secondary") protein which is the real antiviral agent (BARON et al., 1966). These workers suggest that maintenance of stable antiviral activity in the presence of interferon may be due to the continued production of enough antiviral protein (secondary) to balance its loss by decay. The system thus appears to consist of two distinct proteins.

The activity of interferon requires the formation of DNA-dependent RNA, since it can be suppressed by inhibiting the synthesis of both RNA and protein. Probably interferon derepresses a host gene, so leading to the formation of new messenger RNA and hence new protein (SONNABEND and FRIEDMANN, 1966); this postulated new protein would be the effective antiviral agent. As BARON and LEVY (1966) have pointed out, however, the new RNA could be this new antiviral substance. In this manner, very small amounts of interferon would lead to the formation of a large amount of antiviral substance; this seems to be true in practice. If interferon is removed from contact with the cells after a time, then the antiviral action continues for some while afterwards (SONNABEND and FRIEDMANN, 1966).

LEVY et al. (1966) consider that the action of interferon takes place very soon after viral infection. It does not affect adsorption, penetration or uncoating; its action occurs after uncoating but before the formation of viral polyribosomes. LEVY and CARTER (1966) consider that the evidence available indicates that the antiviral action occurs so early as to suggest that the infecting virus particle itself may be involved as the focus. They have shown that the parental RNA of Mengo virus never attaches to the ribosomal sub-unit, but that a pseudopolysome is formed which is scarcely able to synthesise viral RNA and viral protein, or viral RNA-polymerase. Such ribosomes, however, continue to bind and translate cellular messenger RNA. OHNO and NOZIMA (1964) and GOSH and GIFFORD (1965) have shown that in poxvirus-infected cells the rise of such enzymes as thymidine kinase is suppressed; at the same time, the early rise in cytoplasmic RNA fails to take place (OHNO and NOZIMA, 1964).

JOKLIK (1968) found that the secondary protein blocks the formation of polyribosomes in vaccinia-infected L-cells pretreated with interferon. A reduced level of RNA polymerase has been reported by SONNABEND et al. (1967) in chick cells infected with Semliki Forest virus.

SONNABEND and FRIEDMANN (1966) have suggested that the target of interferon may be viral messenger RNA, and that the apparent immunity of host cell protein synthesis may be due to either (a) possession of characteristic structural features of viral as against cell messenger RNA leading to distinctive recognition or (b) differences in the mechanism of protein synthesis or ribosomes when directed by viral RNA. It prevents the parental single strand of viral RNA from being incorporated into the ribonuclease-resistant 2-stranded form which is presumably the replicative state (FINTER, 1966). Thus it seems that interferon blocks the translation of viral RNA into protein, but does not interfere with the transcription of RNA from DNA (DE SOMER and COCITO, 1968).

In regard to oncogenic viruses, TODARO and BARON (1965) have reported inhibition of the transformation of mouse 3T3 cells by SV40 virus by interferon. TAKEMOTO and BARON (1966) have demonstrated viral resistance which is apparently not genetic in origin.

In view of the species specificity, the most promising approach to the treatment of human viral diseases would seem to be through the production of interferon in human cells. There are two possible ways in which this might be done. One is the production in bulk in tissue culture of human diploid cells (CHANY et al., 1968). The other is the induction of interferon in each individual patient. Both statolon and helenine are capable of stimulating the synthesis of interferon.

The isolation of statolon from cultures of Penicillium stoloniferum was reported by KLEINSCHMIDT and PROBST (1962). This substance was originally described as M5-8450 by POWELL et al. (1952). It was shown to inhibit the growth of virus in tissue culture, in animals (KLEINSCHMIDT et al., 1964) and in birds and there is no doubt that it exerts its antiviral action through the synthesis of interferon (KLEINSCHMIDT et al., 1964; KLEINSCHMIDT and Murphy, 1965).

In chickens, a relatively high molecular weight interferon (M.W. 110,000) is produced soon after injection of statolon and this is followed by the production of a lighter interferon (M.W. 30,000) later on (MERIGAN, 1967 b). This latter type of interferon cannot be distinguished from that induced by viral infection.

In mice, optimal protection against viral infection is obtained when statolon is given intraperitoneally 24 hours before the virus (POWELL et al., 1952). The peak level of interferon production occurs about twelve hours after injection of statolon (KLEINSCHMIDT and MURPHY, 1967); there is a direct relationship between the amount of interferon synthesised and the amount of statolon given when the latter is in the lower dose range; however, at a certain point and beyond, the induction of interferon is maximal.

WHEELOCK (1967) has reported that statolon inhibits leukaemia in mice when given as early as six days before or as late as seven days after inoculation of Friend virus. Most of the mice become completely resistant to subsequent challenge by this virus.

The presence of interferon in cells limits the production of more interferon and there is no further formation until the concentration has fallen to minimal amounts (KLEINSCHMIDT and MURPHY, 1967). Hyporeactivity to a second dose of statolon lasts for five to six days as with other agents which induce the formation of interferon.

The active substance was formerly thought to be a polyanionic polysaccharide; however, recent work points firmly to RNA.

ELLIS and KLEINSCHMIDT (1967) and KLEINSCHMIDT et al. (1968) have studied the partially-purified material by electron microscopy and found that it, and also the mycelium, contain particles of typical viral morphology. These particles are hexagonal in shape, about 30 mμ diameter, and their presence is associated with the interferon-inducing fraction of the material. A second fraction which also carries interferon-inducing activity did not contain these particles, however. It appears that this is the first time that viruses have been found in association with fungi imperfecti, and ELLIS and KLEINSCHMIDT (1967) point out that fungal viruses may not be so rare as is supposed KLEINSCHMIDT et al. (1968) find the viral particles to be associated with double-stranded RNA.

Further support for the idea that a virus is responsible for the interferon-inducing capacity of statolon is given by BANKS et al. (1968). These workers have isolated a virus from cultures of P. stoloniferum strain ATCC 14586, and have also put forward evidence which indicates that the active component of statolon is double-stranded viral RNA. BANKS et al. (1968) examined six strains of P. stoloniferum other than ATCC 14586 but found neither virus nor interferon-stimulating activity in extracts of these strains. Elimination of virus from the ATCC 14586 organism by heat-treatment resulted in the loss of interferon-induction.

At the same time, the presence of a polyhedral virus in cultures of a strain of Penicillium funiculosum has also been observed. This latter species of Penicillium yields the antiviral agent helenine (SHOPE, 1953 a, b). LEWIS et al. (1959) had already reported that the antiviral moiety of helenine bore the properties of a ribonucleo-protein. As with statolon, the activity of helenine stems from its induction of interferon (RYTEL, SHOPE and KILBOURNE, 1966; SHOPE, 1966).

FIELD et al. (1967) have reported the induction of interferon by a small amount of double-stranded RNA derived from Escherichia coli infected with coliphage MS 2, and the same group found a double-stranded form of RNA, probably of viral origin, in helenine (LAMPSON et al., 1967). They point out that earlier reports of induction of interferon by DNA and single-stranded RNA involved very large amounts of nucleic acid.

There is good reason to believe, therefore, that both statolon and helenine contain viruses which form double-stranded RNA for their nucleic acid, furthermore, that this induces the production of interferon and is therefore responsible for the antiviral activity of these preparations.

Thus it now seems that double- or multi-stranded RNA, of diverse origins, is capable of inducing interferon formation. FIELD et al. (1967) showed that the single-stranded RNA obtained from the same coliphage used for production of the double-stranded form was inactive even when used in 100 µg doses in rabbits whereas the double-stranded form was active in doses of the order of 1 µg. In the meantime, MERIGAN (1967 a) quoting joint work with Regelson, reported that a plastic, pyran copolymer, can induce the formation of interferon in man. Pyran itself is apparently unsuitable for clinical use as it is pyrogenic and accumulates in the tissues, but the observation opens the way for further investigation of this class of materials. From many points of view, though particularly from that of production, the use of synthetic molecules is an attractive alternative to that of naturally-occurring molecules. Recently DE CLERCQ and MERIGAN (1969) have reported a study on the relative efficiency of various molecules of this class as interferon inducers.

However, the idea that double-stranded synthetic polynucleotides actually induces the synthesis of interferon is challenged by YOUNGNER and HALLUM (1968) who present evidence indicating that a release of preformed material is more likely. In their experiments, the appearance of interferon in mice given double-stranded polyribo-inosinic acid: polyribocytidylic acid heteropolymer was not prevented by blockade of protein synthesis with cycloheximide.

That the use of these synthetic molecules may not be confined to "straight-forward" virus infections is indicated by RHIM et al. (1969) who showed that poly-rI: poly-rC has an inhibitory effect on murine leukaemia and sarcoma viruses in cell cultures. It is clearly impossible at this stage to forecast the possible use of this type of agent in the control of naturally-occurring virus-induced tumours and in particular of human cancer. Nevertheless, it will be recalled that LEVY et al. (1969) studied the effect of poly-rI: poly-rC on a variety of solid tumours and leukaemia in mice, and reported increased survival times of the animals, decreased growth rate of tumours and regression of some established tumours. These neoplasms were not known to contain infectious virus although that induced by adenovirus type 12 contained the T-antigen. It is unlikely that the effects were due solely, if at all, to the induction of interferon. The authors suggest the possibilities of enhanced immune response, direct action of the heteropolymer on the tumour perhaps through ribosomes, or a change in blood supply with subsequent necrosis.

In summary, it now seems more likely that interferon inducers, rather than interferon itself, will be the most appropriate target for practical use (HILLEMAN, 1968; MERIGAN, 1967 c). Such inducers may be either double- or poly-stranded RNA molecules or synthetic polymers resembling these since the double-stranded form of RNA is, at least, by far the most efficient form of naturally-occurring nucleic acid for induction of interferon. In clinical practice, it seems at this stage that the use of interferon-inducers will develop as a prophylactic rather than a therapeutic method.

References

ACORNLEY, J. E., BESSELL, C. J., BYNOE, M. L., GODTFREDSEN, W. O., KNOYLE, J. M.: Antiviral activity of sodium fusidate and related compounds. Brit. J. Pharmacol. 31, 210 (1967).

ADAMSON, R. H., HART, L. G., DE VITA, V. T., OLIVERIO, V. T.: Antitumour activity and some pharmacological properties of anthramycin methyl ester. Cancer Res. 28, 343 (1968).

AISENBERG, A. C., WILKES, B.: Studies on the suppression of immune responses by the periwinkle alkaloids vincristine and vinblastine. J. clin. Invest. 43, 2394 (1964).

ALEXANDER, C. S., NAGASAWA, H. T.: Aminonucleoside of puromycin: elimination of nephrotoxicity by acetylation of the aminoribose moiety. Biochem. Pharmacol. 13, 548 (1964).

ALEXANDER, P., DELORME, E. J., HAMILTON, L. D. G., HALL, J. G.: Effect of nucleic acids from immune lymphocytes on rat sarcomata. Nature (Lond.) 213, 569 (1967).

ALLEN, D. W., ZAMECNIK, P. C.: The effect of puromycin on rabbit reticulocyte ribosomes. Biochim. biophys. Acta (Amst.) 55, 865 (1962).

ANDERTON, K., RICKARDS, R. W.: Some structural features of borrelidin, an antiviral antibiotic. Nature (Lond.) 206, 269 (1965).

ANSFIELD, F. J.: Phase I study of azotomycin (NSC 56654). Cancer Chemother. Rep. 46, 37 (1965).

AOKI, T., BOYSE, E. A., OLD, L. J.: Occurrence of natural antibody to the G (Gross) leukaemia antigen in mice. Cancer Res. 26, 1415 (1966).

APFEL, C. A., ARNASON, B. G., PETERS, J. H.: Induction of tumour immunity with tumour cells treated with iodoacetate. Nature (Lond.) 209, 694 (1966).

ARISON, R. N., FENDALE, E. L.: Induction of renal tumours by streptozotocin in rats. Nature (Lond.) 214, 1254 (1967).

ARLINGHAUS, R., MORRIS, A., FAVELUKES, S., SCHWEST, R.: Effect of puromycin on haemoglobin synthesis. Fed. Proc. 21, 412 (1962).

ARMSTRONG, J. G.: The mechanism of action of the vinca alkaloids. In: Cancer Chemotherapy. Eds.: I. BRODSKY, S. B. KHAN, and J. H. MOYER. London-New York: Grune & Stratton 1967, pp. 37—45.

—, DYKE, R. W., FONTS, P. J., HAWTHORNE, J. J., JANSEN, C. J., JR., PEABODY, A. M.: Initial clinical experience with vinglycinate sulphate, a molecular modification of vinblastine. Cancer Res. 27, 221 (1967).

ASHESHOV, I. N., STRELITZ, F., HALL, E. A., FLON, H.: Survey of actinomycetes for antiphage activity. Antibiot. Chemother. 4, 380 (1953).

AURELIAN, L., ROIZMAN, B.: Abortive infection of canine cells by herpes simplex virus. II. Alternative suppression of synthesis of interferon and viral constituents. J. mol. Biol. 11, 539 (1965).

BACK, N., AMBRUS, J. L., KLEIN, E., MILGROM, H., VELASCO, H., AUSMAN, R. K., STUTZMAN, L., SOKAL, J. E.: Systemic and local antitumour effect of the antibiotic spiramycin: a pharmacologic and clinical study. Acta Unio intern. contra Cancrum 20, 300 (1964).

BAKER, B. R., SCHAUB, R. E., JOSEPH, J. P., WILLIAMS, J. H.: Puromycin. Synthetic studies. IX. Total synthesis. J. Amer. Chem. Soc. 77, 12 (1955).

BALANDIN, I. G., MELNIKOVA, L. A., KOZLOVA, I. A., PETERSON, O. P., MASHARINA, L. V., ZHDANOV, V. M.: Action of histone on reproduction of vaccinia virus. Arch. ges. Virusforsch. 18, 350 (1966).

BANKS, G. T., BUCK, K. W., CHAIN, E. B., HIMMELWEIT, F., MARKS, J. E., TYLER, J. M., HOLLINGS, M., LAST, F. T., STONE, O. M.: Viruses in fungi and interferon stimulation. Nature (Lond.) 218, 542 (1968).

BARG, W., BOGGIANO, E., SLOANE, N., DE RENZO, E. C.: Inhibitors of de novo formyl-glycinamide ribotide synthesis in pigeon liver extracts. Fed. Proc. 16, 150 (1957).

BARDOS, T. J., GORDON, H. L., CHMIELEWICZ, Z. F., KUTZ, R. L., NADKARNI, M. V.: A systematic investigation of the presence of growth-inhibitory substances in animal tissues. Cancer Res. 28, 1620—1630 (1968).

BARON, S., BUCKLER, C. E., FRIEDMAN, R. M., McCLOSKEY, R. V.: Role of interferon during viraemia. II. Protective action of circulating interferon. J. Immunol. 96, 17 (1966).

—, LEVY, H. B.: Interferon. Ann. Rev. Microbiol. 20, 291 (1966).

BARSKI, G., CORNEFERT, F.: Response of different mouse cell strains to polyoma infection in vitro. Latency and self-inhibitory effect in infected cultures. J. nat. Cancer Inst. 28, 823 (1962).

BAUER, D. J.: Possible correlation between virus particle size and activity of antiviral agents. Nature (Lond.) 209, 639 (1966).

BECKER, J., DANIEL, J. W., RUSCH, H. P.: Growth inhibition of Physarum polycephalum for the evaluation of chemotherapeutic agents. Cancer Res. 23, 1910 (1963).

BENNETTE, J. G.: Isolation of a non-pathogenic tumour-destroying virus from mouse ascites. Nature (Lond.) 182, 72 (1960).

BEN-PORAT, T., REISSIG, M., KAPLAN, A. S.: Effect of mitomycin C on the synthesis of infective virus and deoxribonucleic acid in pseudorabies virus-infected rabbit kidney cells. Nature (Lond.) 190, 33 (1961).

BERGSAGEL, D. E., ROSS, S. W., DAVIS, P.: Evaluation of new chemotherapeutic agents in the treatment of multiple myeloma. II. Mitomycin C (NSC-26980). Cancer Chemother. Rep. 21, 75 (1962).

BERLIN, Y. A., CHUPRUNOVA, O. A., KLYASHCHITSKII, B. A. et al.: Olivomycin. 3. The structure of olivomycin. Tetrahedron Lett. 14, 1425 (1966).

BERNARD, J., JACQUILLAT, C., BOIRON, M., NAJCAN, Y., SELIGMANN, M., TANZER, J., WEIL, M., LORTHOLARY, P.: Essai de traitement des leucemies aigues lymphoblastoques et myeloblastiques par un antibiotique nouveau: la rubidomycine (13 057 RP). Etude de 61 observations. Presse med. 75, 951 (1967).

BHUYAN, B. K.: Pactamycin, an antibiotic that inhibits protein synthesis. Biochem. Pharmacol. 16, 1410 (1967).

—, DIETZ, A.: Fermentation, taxonomic and biological studies of Nogalomycin. Antimicrobial Agents and Chemotherapy, 1965. Ed.: GLADYS L. HOBBY. Amer. Soc. Microbiol. 1965, pp. 836—844.

— —, SMITH, C. G.: Pactamycin, a new anti-tumour biotic. I. Discovery and biological properties. Antimicrobial Agents and Chemotherapy, 1961. Ed.: GLADYS L. HOBBY. Amer. Soc. Microbiol. 1961, pp. 184—190.

—, JOHNSON, R. L.: Metabolic studies of pactamycin. Biochem. Pharmacol. 12, 1001 (1963).

—, RENIS, H. E., SMITH, C. G.: A collagen-plate assay for cytotoxic agents. II. Biological studies. Cancer Res. 22, 1131 (1962).

—, SMITH, C. G.: Differential interaction of nogalomycin with DNA of varying base composition. Proc. nat. Acad. Sci. (U. S.) 54, 566 (1965).

BISMANIS, J. E.: Immunisation of mice against Ehrlich ascites carcinoma with formalized tumour cells grown in tissue culture. J. Path. Bact. 87, 444 (1964).

BOND, W. H., ROBIN, R. J., BATES, L. H., HODES, MARION E.: Treatment of neoplastic diseases with an improved oral preparation of vinblastine sulphate. Cancer 19, 213 (1966).

BORICKY, L., LACKOVIC, V., BLASKOVIC, D., MASLER, L., SUKL, D.: An interferon-like substance induced by mannans. Acta. virol. 11, 264 (1967).

BRADNER, W. T., PINDELL, M. H.: Anti-tumour properties of phleomycin. Nature (Lond.) 196, 682 (1962).

—, SUGIURA, K.: Actinogan: a new antitumour agent obtained from streptomyces. II. Studies with sarcoma 180 and in a tumour spectrum. Cancer Res. 22, 167 (1962).

BROCKMAN, R. W.: Mechanism of resistance to anticancer agents. Advanc. Cancer Res. 7, 129 (1963).

—, ANDERSON, E. P.: Biochemical effects of duazomycin A in the plasma cell neoplasm 70429. Proc. Amer. Ass. Cancer Res. 3, 307 (1962).

BROOME, J. D.: Evidence that the L-asparaginase activity of guinea-pig serum is responsible for its antilymphoma effects. Nature (Lond.) 191, 1114 (1961).
— Evidence that the L-asparaginase of guinea-pig serum is responsible for its antilymphoma effects. I. Properties of the L-asparaginase of guinea-pig serum in relation to those of the antilymphoma substance. J. exp. Med. 118, 99 (1963 a).
— Evidence that the L-asparaginase of guinea-pig serum is responsible for its antilymphoma effects. II. Lymphoma 6C3HED cells cultures in a medium devoid of L-asparaginase lose their susceptibility to the effects of guinea-pig serum in vivo. J. exp. Med. 118, 121 (1963 b).
BROSS, I. D. J., TARNOWSKI, G. S.: A new approach to differential toxicity. Cancer Chemotherapy Screening Data XIII. Cancer Res. 22, 45 (1962).
BROWN, J. H., KENNEDY, B. J.: Mithramycin in the treatment of disseminated testicular neoplasms. New England J. Med. 272, 111 (1965).
BUCKNALL, R. A.: "Species Specificity" of interferons: A misnomer? Nature (Lond.) 216, 1022 (1967).
BULLOUGH, W. S., LAWRENCE, EDNA B.: Epidermal chalone and mitotic control in the Vx2 epidermal tumour. Nature (Lond.) 220, 134 (1968 a).
— — Melanocyte chalone and mitotic control in melanomata. Nature (Lond.) 220, 137 (1968 b).
BURCHENAL, J. H., KREIS, W.: Mechanism of action of antibiotics and new agents. In: Cancer Chemotherapy. Eds.: I. BRODSKY, S. B. KAHN, and J. H. MOYER. London: Grune & Stratton 1967, p. 46.
—, OETTGEN, H. F., REPPART, J. A., COLEY, V.: The effect of actinomycins and their derivatives on a spectrum of transplanted mouse leukaemia. Ann. N. Y. Acad. Sci. 89, 399 (1960).
BÜRK, R. R.: Wistar Inst. Symp. Monogr. No. 7 (1967), p. 39.
BURKITT, D.: African lymphoma. Observations on the response to vincristine sulphate therapy. Cancer 19, 1131 (1966).
Cancer Chemotherapy National Service Centre: An outline of procedures for preliminary toxicologic and pharmacologic evaluation of experimental cancer chemotherapeutic agents. Cancer Chemother. Rep. 37, 1 (1964).
CAREY, R. W., HOLLAND, J. F., WHANG, H. Y., NETER, E., BRYANT, B.: Clostridial oncolysis in man. Europ. J. Cancer 3, 37 (1967).
CARTER, S. B.: Action of cytochalasins. Nature (Lond.) 213, 261 (1967).
CARVER, D. H., NAFICY, K.: Inhibition of arbor viruses (Group A) by a protein-like constituent of a corynebacterium. Proc. Soc. exp. Biol. (N. Y.) 111, 356 (1962).
— — Studies on viral inhibitors of biological origin. I. Inhibition of viral replication by protein-like constituents of bacteria. Proc. Soc. exp. Biol. (N. Y.) 116, 548 (1964).
—, ROSEN, F. S.: Viral inhibitors of biological origin. II. A viral inhibitory factor obtained from E. coli O.III and inhibition of viral replication by nucleic acid derivatives. Proc. Soc. exp. Biol. (N. Y.) 116, 575 (1964).
CASAZZA, A. M., GHIONE, M.: Therapeutic action of distamycin A on vaccinia virus infection in vivo. Chemotherapia 9, 80 (1964).
CASSEL, W. A., GARRETT, R. E.: Relationship between viral neurotropism and oncolysis. I. Study of vaccinia virus. Cancer 20, 433 (1967 a).
— — Relationship between viral neurotropism and oncolysis. II. Study of influenza virus. Cancer 20, 440 (1967 b).
CENTIFANTO, YSOLINA M.: A therapeutic anticiral from an extract of λ-infected E. coli (Phagicin). Proc. Soc. exp. Biol. (N. Y.) 120, 607 (1965).
— Antiviral agent from λ-infected Escherichia coli K-12. I. Isolation. Appl. Microbiol. 16, 827 (1968).
CERIOTTI, G.: Narciclasine: an antimitotic substance from narcissus bulbs. Nature (Lond.) 213, 595 (1967).
CHANEY, C., FOURNIER, FRANCOISE, FALCOFF, E.: A simple system for the mass production of human interferon: the human amniotic membrane. In: Ciba Foundation Symposium on Interferons. London: Churchill 1968, pp. 64—67.
CHIRIGOS, M. A.: Studies with the murine leukaemogenic Rauscher virus. III. An in vivo assay for anti-viral agents. Cancer Res. 24, 1035 (1964).

54 References

Coffee, G. L., Hillegas, A. B., Knudsen, M. P., Koepsell, H. J., Oyaas, J. E., Ehrlich, J.: Azaserine: microbiological studies. Antibiot. Chemother. 4, 775 (1954).

Cohen, A., Harley, E. H., Rees, K. R.: Antiviral effect of daunomycin. Nature (Lond.) 222, 36 (1969).

Cohen, M. M., Shaw, M. M., Craig, A. P.: The effects of streptonigrin on cultured human leucocytes. Proc. nat. Acad. Sci. (U.S.) 50, 16 (1963).

Cohen, R. A., Kucera, L. S., Hermann, E. C., Jr.: Antiviral activity of Melissa officinalis (lemon balm) extract. Proc. Soc. exp. Biol. (N. Y.) 117, 431 (1964)

Colombo, B., Felicetti, L., Baglioni, C.: Inhibition of protein synthesis by cycloheximide in rabbit reticulocytes. Biochem. Biophys. Res. Commun. 18, 389 (1965).

Colon, J. I., Idoine, Jane B., Brand, O. M., Costlow, R. D.: Mode of action of an inhibitor from agar on growth and haemagglutination of group A arboviruses. J. Bact. 90, 172 (1965).

Cooke, P. M., Stevenson, J. W.: Antiviral substance from Penicillium cyaneo-fulvum Biourge. I. Production and partial purification. Canad. J. Microbiol. 11, 913 (1965 a).

— — Antiviral substance from Penicillium cyaneo-fulvum Biourge. II. Biological activities against RNA-containing viruses. Canad. J. Microbiol. 11, 921 (1965 b).

Creasey, W. A.: Antitumoral activity of the fern Cibotium schiedei. Nature (Lond.) 222, 1281 (1969).

Curreri, A. R., Ansfield, F. K.: Mithramycin—human toxicology and preliminary therapeutic investigation. Cancer Chemother. Rep. 8, 18 (1960).

Cutting, W., Furusawa, S., Woo, Y. K.: Antiviral activity of herbs on Columbia SK in mice, and LCM, vaccinia and adeno type 12 viruses in vitro. Proc. Soc. exp. Biol. (N. Y.) 120, 330 (1965).

Dafni, Z., Chilo, M.: Cytotoxic principle of the phytoflagellate Pyrmnesium parvum. J. Cell. Biol. 28, 461 (1966).

David-West, T. S., Cooke, Patricia M., Stevenson, J. W.: New methods of production and partial purification of an antiviral substance from Penicillium cyaneo-fulvum. Canad. J. Microbiol. 14, 189 (1968 a).

— — — The mode of action of an antiviral substance from Penicillium cyaneo-fulvum. Canad. J. Microbiol. 14, 197 (1968 b).

de Clercq, E., Merigan, T. C.: Requirement of a stable secondary structure for the antiviral activity of polynucleotides. Nature (Lond.) 222, 1148 (1969).

Dederick, M. M., Nevinny, H. B., Hall, T. C., Potee, K. G.: Preliminary report on human toxicity study of streptovitacin A. Cancer Chemother. Rep. 27, 81 (1963).

Delta, B. G., Pinkel, D., Magtibay, L., Hubbard, J.: Streptovitacin A in children with cancer. Cancer Chemother. Rep. 11, 45 (1961).

Desmyter, J., Rawls, W. E., Melnick, J. L.: A human interferon that crosses the species line. Proc. nat. Acad. Sci. (Wash.) 59, 69 (1968).

De Somer, P., Cocito, C.: The mode of action of interferon. In: Ciba Foundation Symposium on Interferons. London: Churchill 1968, p. 128 et seq.

De Voe, S. E., Rigler, N. E., Shay, A. J., Martin, J. H., Boyd, T. C., Backus, E. J., Mowat, J. H., Bohonos, N.: Alazopeptin: production, isolation and chemical characteristics. Antibiot. Ann., pp. 730—735 (1957).

Dice, J. W., Rightsel, W. A., Schabel, F. M., Jr., McLean, I. W., Jr.: Experiences in developing potential antiviral compounds. Ann. N. Y. Acad. Sci. 130, 24 (1965).

Dickinson, Lois, Griffiths, A. J., Mason, C. G., Mills, R. F. N.: Antiviral activity of two antibiotics isolated from a species of Streptomyces. Nature (Lond.) 206, 265 (1965).

Dickson, J. A.: Tissue-culture approach to the treatment of cancer. Brit. med. J. 1, 817 (1966).

Dijkman, N. J., Boss, M. L., Lichter, W., Sigel, M. M., O'Connor, J. E., Search, N.: Cytotoxic substances from tropical plants. Chemotherapy Screening Data XLVIII. Cancer Res. 26, 1121 (1966).

Di Marco, A., Gaetani, M., Orezzi, P., Scarpinato, B. M., Silvestrini, R., Soldati, M., Dasdia, T., Valentini, L.: Daunomycin, a new antibiotic of the rhodomycin group. Nature (Lond.) 201, 706 (1964 a).

— —, Dorigotti, L., Soldat, M., Bellini, O.: Daunomycin: a new antibiotic with antitumour activity. Cancer Chemother. Rep. 38, 31 (1964 b).

DIMARCO, A., SOLDATI, M., FIORETTI, A., DASDIA, T.: Activity of daunomycin, a new antitumour antibiotic, on normal and neoplastic cells grown in vitro. Cancer Chemother. Rep. 38, 39 (1964 c).

DI MARCO, P., GAETANI, M., OREZZI, P., SCOTTI, T., ARCAMONE, F.: Experimental studies on distamycin A—a new antibiotic with cytotoxic activity. Chemother. Rep. 18, 15 (1962).

DION, H. W., FUSARI, S. A., JACUBOWSKI, Z. L., ZORA, J. G., BARTZ, Q. R.: 6-diazo-5-oxo-L-norleucine, a new tumour-inhitory substance. II. Isolation and characterisation. J. Amer. Chem. Soc. 78, 3075 (1956).

DI PAOLO, J. A., MOORE, G. E.: An evaluation of ascites tumour cell plating for screening chemotherapeutic agents. Antibiot. Chemotherapy 7, 465 (1957).

—, TARBELL, D. S., MOORE, G. E.: Studies on the carcinolytic activity of fumagillin and some of its derivates. Antibiot. Ann. 1959, pp. 541—546.

DJORDJEVIC, B., KIM, J. H.: Lethal effect of phleomycin in different stages of the division cycle of HeLa cells. Cancer Res. 27, 2255 (1967).

DOLOWY, W. V., CORNET, J., HENSON, D., AMMERAAL, R.: Response of intercerebral Gardner lymphosarcoma to guinea-pig L-asparaginase and E. coli L-asparaginase. Proc. Soc. exp. Biol. (N. Y.) 123, 133 (1966).

DORFMAN, R. I.: Inhibition of tumour growth by steroids. In: Methods in Hormone Research. Ed.: R. I. DORFMAN. New York: Academic Press 1965, Vol. 4, Pt. B, pp. 165—192.

DUBACH, U. C.: Aminonucleosid-nephrose. Progr. Drug. Res. 7, 340 (1964).

DUBOST, M., GANTER, P., MARAL, R., NINET, L., PINNERT, S., PREUD'HOMME, J., WERNER, G. H.: Un nouvel antibiotique à propriétés cytostatique: la rubidomycine. Compt. rend. Acad Sci. 257, 1813 (1963).

DUTCHER, J. D., VON SALTZA, M. H., PANSY, F. E.: Septacidin, a new antitumour and antifungal antibiotic produced by Streptomyces fimbriatus. Antimicrobial Agents Chemotherapy 1963, pp. 83—88.

DUVALL, L. R.: 6-diazo-5-oxo-norleucine. Cancer Chemother. Rep. 7, 86 (1960).

— Porfiromycin. Cancer Chemother. Rep. 30, 35 (1963).

EAGLE, H., FOLEY, G. E.: The cytotoxic action of carcinolytic agents in tissue culture. Amer. J. Med. 21, 739 (1956).

— — Susceptibility of cultured human cells to antitumour agents. Ann. N. Y. Acad. Sci. 76, 534 (1958).

EDERY, H., SCHATZBERG-PORATH, G., GITTER, S.: Pharmacodynamic activity of elatericin (cucurbitacin D). Arch. int. Pharmacodyn. 130, 315 (1960).

EHRLICH, J. ANDERSON, L. E., COFFEY, G. L., HILLEGAS, A. B., KNUDSEN, M. P., KOEPSELL, H. J., KOHBERGER, D. L., OYAAS, J. E.: Antibiotic studies of azaserine. Nature (Lond.) 173, 72 (1954).

—, COFFEY, G. L., FISHER, M. W., HILLEGAS, A. B., KOHBERGER, D. L., MACHAMER, H. E., RIGHTSEL, W. A., ROEGNER, F. R.: 6-diazo-5-oxo-L-norleucine, a new tumour inhibitory substance. I. Biologic studies. Antibiot. Chemother. 6, 487 (1956).

—, SLOAN, B. J., MILLER, F. A., MACHAMER, H. E.: Searching for antiviral materials from microbial fermentations. Ann. N. Y. Acad. Sci. 130, 5 (1965).

EL-AMMAR, F. A., GREENBERG, D. M.: Studies on the mechanism of inhibition of tumour growth by the enzyme glutaminase. Cancer Res. 26, 116 (1966).

ELION, G. B., HITCHINGS, G.: Metabolic basis for the actions of analogues of purine and pyrimidines. Advanc. Chemotherapy 2, 91 (1965).

ELLIS, L. F., KLEINSCHMIDT, T. J.: Virus-like particles of a fraction of statolon, a mould product. Nature (Lond.) 215, 649 (1967).

ELLISON, ROSE R.: Preliminary clinical trials of hadacidin, a new tumour-inhibitory substance. Clin. Pharmacol. Therap. 4, 326 (1963).

— Clinical pharmacologic study of hadacidin (NSC-521778). Cancer Chemother. Rep. 46, 31—36 (1965).

EMMELOT, P.: The molecular basis of cancer chemotherapy. In: Molecular Pharmacology, Vol. 2. Ed.: E. J. ARIENS. New York: Academic Press 1965, pp. 53—198.

ENDO, H., ISHIZAWA, M., KAMIYA, T., SONODA, S.: Relation between tumoricidal and prophage-inducing action. Nature (Lond.) 198, 258 (1963).

ENGELBART, K., GERICKE, D.: Oncolysis by Clostridia. V. Transplanted tumours of the hamster; extensive or complete lysis of tumour. Cancer Res. 24, 239 (1964).

ESPENSHADE, M. A., GRIFFITH, E. M.: Tumour-inhibiting Basidiomycetes, isolation and cultivation in the laboratory. Mycologia 58, 511 (1966).

EVANS, A. E.: Mitomycin C. Cancer Chemother. Rep. 14, 1 (1961).

— Chemotherapy of solid tumours in children. In: Cancer Chemotherapy. Eds.: I. BRODSKY, S. B. KHAN and J. H. MOYER. New York: Grune & Stratton 1967, pp. 133—139.

EVANS, J. S., MENGEL, G. D., CERU, J., JOHNSTON, R. L.: Biological studies on streptovitacin A, a new antitumour agent. Antibiot. Ann. 1959, pp. 565—571.

FALASCHI, A., KORNBERG, A.: Phleomycin, an inhibitor of DNA polymerase. Fed. Proc. 23, Pt. I, 940 (1964).

FALKE, D., KOHLHAGE, H., NIESSING, K.: Effect of actidione on the synthesis of herpes simplex virus in cultures of various cell types. Z. Naturforsch. B. 21, 447 (1966).

FANTES, K. H.: Further purification of chick interferon. Nature (Lond.) 207, 1298 (1965).

— Purification, concentration and physicochemical properties of interferons. In: Interferons. Ed.: N. B. FINTER. Amsterdam: North-Holland Publishing Co. 1966, pp. 119—180.

FARBER, S.: Clinical and biological studies with the actinomycins. In: Ciba Foundation Symposium on Amino Acids, Peptides and Antimetabolic Activity. London: Churchill 1959, pp. 138—148.

—, D'ANGIO, G., EVANS, A., MITUS, A.: Clinical studies of actinomycin D with special reference to Wilms' tumour in children. Ann. N. Y. Acad. Sci. 89, 421 (1960).

FERGUSON, D., HUMPHREY, E.: Mitomycin C. (Preliminary trial note.) Cancer Chemother. Rep. 8, 154 (1960).

FERNBACH, D. J., MARTYN, D. T.: Role of dactinomycin in the improved survival of children with Wilms' tumour. J. Amer. med. Ass. 195, 1005 (1966).

FIELD, A. K., LAMPSON, G. P., TYTELL, A. A., NEMES, M. M., HILLEMAN, M. R.: Inducers of interferon and host resistance. IV. Double-stranded replicative form RNA (MS2-RF-RNA) from E. coli infected with MS2 coliphage. Proc. nat. Acad. Sci. (Wash.) 58, 2102 (1967).

FIELD, J. B.: Clinical evaluation of streptovitacin A. Cancer Chemother. Rep. 31, 53 (1963).

—, COSTA, F., BORYCZKA, A.: Origin of a new antitumour agent, streptovitacin. Antibiot. Ann. 1959, pp. 547—550.

FINKELSTEIN, R. A.: Alteration of susceptibility of embryonated eggs to Newcastle disease virus by Escherichia coli and endotoxin. Proc. Soc. exp. Biol. Med. (N. Y.) 106, 481 (1961).

FINTER, N. B.: Interferon assays and standards. In: Interferons. Ed.: N. B. FINTER. Amsterdam: North-Holland Publishing Co. 1966, pp. 87—118.

FITZGERALD, D. B., HARTWELL, J. L., LEITER, J.: Tumour-damaging activity in plant families showing antimalarial activity: Amaryllidaceae. J. nat. Cancer Inst. 20, 763 (1958).

FOLEY, G. E., EPSTEIN, S. S.: Cell culture and cancer chemotherapy. Advanc. Chemotherapy 1, 175 (1964).

—, McCARTHY, R. E., BINNS, V. M., SNELL, E. E., GUIRARD, B. M., KIDDER, G. V., DEWEY, V. C., THAYER, P. S.: A comparative study of the use of micro-organisms in the screening of potential antiviral agents. Ann. N. Y. Acad. Sci. 76, 413 (1958).

FOULDS, L.: The experimental study of tumour progression: a review. Cancer Res. 14, 327 (1954).

FRANKLIN, R. M.: The inhibition of ribonucleic acid synthesis in mammalian cells by actinomycin D. Biochem. biophys. Acta 12, 555 (1963).

FREED, J. J., SOROF, S.: Reversible inhibition of cell multiplication by a small class of liver proteins. Biochem. Biophys. Res. Commun. 22, 1 (1966).

FREI, E., WHANG, JACQUELINE, SCOGGINS, R. B., VAN SCOTT, E. J., RALL, D. P., BEN, M.: The stathmokinetic effect of vincristine. Cancer Res. 24, 1918 (1964).

FRENCH, T. C., DAWID, I. B., DAY, R. A., BUCHANAN, J. M.: Azaserine-reactive sulfhydryl group of 2-formamido-N-ribosylacetamide-5'-phosphate: L-glutamine amidoligase (adenosine diphosphate). I. Purification and properties of the enzyme from Salmonella typhimurium and the synthesis of L-azaserine-C14. J. biol. Chem. 238, 2171 (1963).

FRIEDMAN, R. M., PASTAN, IRA: Specific inhibition of virus growth in cells treated with phospholipase C. Proc. nat. Acad. Sci. 59, 1371 (1968).

FRUITSTONE, M. J., WADDELL, G. H., SIGEL, M. M.: An interferon produced in response to infection by herpes simplex virus. Proc. Soc. exp. Biol. Med. (N. Y.) 117, 804 (1964).

FURUZAWA, CUTTING, W.: Antiviral activity of higher plants on lymphocytic choriomeningitis infection in vitro and in vivo. Proc. Soc. exp. Biol. (N. Y.) 122, 280 (1966).

GALE, G. R., SCHMIDT, G. B.: Mode of action of alanosine. Biochem. Pharmacol. 17, 363 (1968).

GALLILLY, R., SHOHAT, B., KALISH, J., GITTER, S., LAVIE, D.: Further studies on the antitumour effect of cucurbatacins. Cancer Res. 22, 1038 (1962).

GARATTINI, S., SPROSTON, E. M. (eds.): Antitumoural effects of Vinca rosea alkaloids. Proc. 1st Symp. G.E.C.A. (Groupe Europeen de Chimiothérapie anticancereuse, Paris, June 1965). Amsterdam: Excerpta Medica Foundation 1966.

GARD, S.: Vaccines against viral and rickettsial diseases of man. Brit. med. J. 2, 1590 (1966).

GARREN, L. D., HOWELL, R. R., TOMKINS, G. M., GROCCO, R. M.: A paradoxical effect of actinomycin D: the mechanism of regulation of enzyme synthesis of hydrocortisone. Proc. nat. Acad. Sci. (U. S.) 52, 1121 (1964).

GAUSE, G. F.: Olivomycin, mithramycin, chromomycin. Three related cancerostatic antibiotics. Advan. Chemotherapy 2, 179 (1965).

— Microbial models of cancer cells. Amsterdam: North-Holland Publishing Co. 1966.

—, KOTCHETKOVA, G. V., VLADIMIROVA, G. V.: Action of anticancer substances on the biochemical mutants of microorganisms with impaired oxidation. Cancer Chemother. Rep. 4, 48 (1959).

GELDERMAN, A. H., LINCOLN, T. L., COWIE, D. B., ROBERTS, B.: A further correlation between the response of lysogenic bacteria and tumour cells to chemical agents. Proc. nat. Acad. Sci. (U. S.) 55, 289 (1966).

GELLERT, M., SMITH, C. E., NEVILLE, D., FELSENFIELD, G.: Actinomycin binding to DNA; mechanism and specificity. J. mol. Biol. 11, 445 (1965).

GELLHORN, A., HIRSCHBERG, E. (Eds.): Investigation of diverse systems for cancer chemotherapy screening. Cancer Res. 1955, Suppl. 3.

GEORGE, P., JOURNEY, L. J., GOLDSTEIN, M. N.: Effect of vincristine on the fine structure of HeLa cells during mitosis. J. nat. Cancer Inst. 35, 355 (1965).

GERICKE, D., ENGELBART, K.: Oncolysis by Clostridia. II. Experiments on a tumour spectrum with a variety of clostridia in combination with heavy metals. Cancer Res. 24, 217 (1964).

GIFFORD, G. E., HELLER, E.: Effect of actinomycin D on interferon production by "active" and "inactive" Chikungunya virus in chick cells. Nature (Lond.) 200, 50 (1963).

GILDEN, R. V., CARP, R. I.: Effects of cycloheximide and puromycin on synthesis of simian virus 40 T-antigen in green monkey kidney cells. J. Bact. 91, 1295 (1966).

GITTERMAN, C. O., DULANEY, E. L., KACZKA, E. A., HENDLIN, D., WOODRUFF, H. B.: The human tumour-egg host system. II. Discovery and properties of a new anti-tumour agent, hadacidin. Proc. Soc. exp. Biol. (N. Y.) 109, 852 (1962).

GLICK, J. L.: The specificity of inhibition of tumour cell viability. Cancer Res. 27, 2338 (1967).

—, GOLDBERG, A. R.: Inhibition of L1210 tumour growth by thymus DNA. Science 149, 997 (1965).

GLYNN, J. P., MOLONEY, J. B., CHIRIGOS, M. A., HUMPHREYS, S. R., GOLDIN, A.: Biological interrelationships in the chemotherapy of Moloney virus leukaemia. Cancer Res. 23, 269 (1963).

GOLD, J.: Metabolic profies in human solid tumours. I. A new technique for the utilisation of human solid tumour cancer research and its application to the anaerobic glycolysis of isologous benign and malignant colon tissues. Cancer Res. 26, 695 (1966).

GOLDBERG, I. H., RABINOWITZ, M.: Actinomycin D. inhibition of deoxyribonucleic acid-dependent synthesis of ribonucleic acid. Science 136, 315 (1962).

—, REICH, E.: Actinomycin inhibition of RNA synthesis directed by DNA. Federation Proc. 23, 958 (1964).

— —, RABINOWITZ, M.: Inhibition of ribonucleic acid-polymerase recations by actinomycin and proflavine. Nature (Lond.) 199, 44 (1963).

GOLDENBERG, I. S.: Vincristine (NSC-67574) therapy of women with advanced breast cancer. Cancer Chemother. Rep. 41, 7 (1964).

GOLDIN, A., VENDITTI, J. M., KLINE, I.: Evaluation of antileukaemic agents and employing advanced leukaemia L.1210 in mice. VI. Cancer Res. **22**, 749 (1962).

GOSH, S. N., GIFFORD, G. E.: Effect of interferon on the dynamics of H3-thymidine incorporation and thymidine kinase induction in chick fibroblast cultures infected with vaccinia virus. Virology **27**, 186 (1965).

GRADY, J. S., LUMMIS, W. L., SMITH, C. G.: Tissue culture bioautographic system. Proc. Soc. exp. Biol. (N. Y.) **103**, 727 (1960).

GRAY, G. D., CAMIENER, G. W., BHUYAN, B. K.: Nogalomycin effects in rat liver. Inhibition of tryptophan pyrrolase induction and nucleic acid biosynthesis. Cancer Res. **26**, 2419 (1966).

GREGORY, F. J., HEALY, E. M., FRANKLIN, S. D., AGERSBORY, H. P. K., JR., WARREN, G. H.: Antitumour activity of Basidiomycete fermentation products. Proc. Amer. Ass. Cancer Res. **7**, 25 (1966) (Abst. 98).

—, RUELIUS, H. W., SCHILLINGS, R. T., FLINT, S. F., WARREN, G. H.: Poricin—an antitumour agent derived from the basidiomycete Poria corticola. Proc. Amer. Ass. Cancer Res. **9**, 26 (1968) (Abst. 100).

GRESSER, I., GROGAN, ELIZABETH A: Inhibition of arboviruses by a constituent of a staphylococcus. Proc. Soc. exp. Biol. (N. Y.) **119**, 1176 (1965).

GRISWOLD, D. P., LASTER, W. R., SNOW, M. Y., SCHABEL, F. M., SKIPPER, H. E.: Experimental evaluation of potential anticancer agents. XII. Quantitative drug response of Sa. 180, Ca. 755 and Leukaemia L.1210 systems to a standard list of active and inactive agents. Cancer Res. **23**, 271 (1963).

GROLLMAN, A.: Inhibitors of protein biosynthesis. II. Mode of action of anisomycin. J. biol. Chem. **242**, 3226 (1967).

GROUPÉ, V., RAUSCHER, F. J.: Response of Rous sarcoma virus to Xerosin (NSC-4927): a microbial product. Cancer Chemother. Rep. **44**, 1 (1965).

HACKENTHAL, C. A., GOLBEY, R. B., TAN, C, T. C., KARNOFSKY, D. A., BURCHENAL, J. H.: Clinical observations on the effects of streptonigrin in patients with neoplastic disease. Antibiot. Chemother. **11**, 178 (1961).

HACKMANN, C.: Experimentelle Untersuchungen über die Wirkung von Actinomycin C (HBF. 396) bei bösartigen Geschwülsten. Z. Krebsforsch. **58**, 607 (1952).

HAFF, R. F.: Inhibition of the multiplication of pseudorabies virus by cycloheximide. Virology **22**, 430 (1964).

HAHON, N., KOZIKOWSKI, E. H.: Induction of interferon by Coxiella burneti in cell cultures. J. gen. Virol. **3**, 125 (1968).

HALL, T. C.: New chemotherapeutic agents in Hodgkin's disease. Cancer Res. **26**, 1297 (1966).

HALPERN, B. N., BIOZZI, G., STIFFEL, C., MONTON, D.: Inhibition of tumour growth by administration of killed Corynebacterium parvum. Nature (Lond.) **212**, 853 (1966).

HALSTEAD, S. B., SUKHAVACHANA, P., NISALAK, A.: Assay of mouse-adapted dengue viruses in mammalian cell cultures by an interference method. Proc. Soc. exp. Biol. (N. Y.) **115**, 1062 (1964).

HANDLER, A. H., SARRIS, T. G., WILLS, C.: Chemotherapy studies on primary tumour grafts and metastases in hamsters and mice. Acta Unio internat. contra Cancrum **20**, 176 (1964).

HANSON, F. R., EBLE, T. E.: An antiphage agent isolated from Aspergillus sp. J. Bact. **58**, 527 (1949).

HARRIS, M. N., MEDREK, T. J., GOLOMB, F. M., GUMPORT, S. L., POSTEL, A. H., WRIGHT, J. C.: Chemotherapy with streptonigrin in advanced cancer. Cancer **18**, 49 (1965).

HARTMANN, G., GOLLER, H., KOSCHEL, K., KERSTEN, W., KERSTEN, H.: Hemmung der DNA-abhängigen RNA- und DNA-Synthese durch Antibiotica. Biochem. Z. **341**, 126 (1964).

HARTWELL, J. L.: Plant remedies for cancer. Cancer Chemother. Rep. **7**, 19 (1960).

HASELKORN, R.: Actinomycin D as a probe for nucleic acid secondary structure. Science **143**, 682 (1964).

HASKELL, C. M., CANELLOS, C. P., LEVENTHAL, B. G., CARBONE, P. P.: L-asparaginase toxicity. Cancer Res. **29**, 974 (1969).

HATA, T.: Antitumour antibiotics from Streptomyces. Acta Unio intern. contra Cancrum **15** (1959), Suppl. 123.

HATA, T., SANO, Y., SUGUWARA, R., MATSUMAE, A., KANAMORI, K. SHIMA, T., HOSHI, T.: Mitomycin, a new antibiotic from Streptomyces. J. Antibiot. (Tokyo) A. 9, 141 (1956).

HECHTER, O., HALKERSTON, I. D. K.: On the action of mammalian hormones. In: The Hormones. Eds.: G. PINCUS, K. V. THIMANN and E. B. ASTWOOD. New York: Academic Press 1964, pp. 607—825.

HELLER, E.: Enhancement of Chikungunya virus replication and inhibition of interferon production by actinomycin D. Virology 21, 652 (1963).

—, ARGAMAN, M., LEVY, H., GOLDBLUM, N.: Selective inhibition of vaccinia virus by the antibiotic rifampicin. Nature (Lond.) 222, 273 (1969).

HENDERSON, J. F., PATERSON, A. R. P., CALDWELL, I. C., HORI, M.: Biochemical effects of formycin, an adenosine analogue. Cancer Res. 27, 715 (1967).

HERMANN, E. C., JR., GABLIKS, J., EAGLE, C., PERLMAN, P. L.: Agar diffusion method for the detection and bioassay of antiviral antibiotics. Proc. Soc. exp. Biol. (N. Y.) 103, 625 (1960).

HERRMANN, R. L., DAY, R. A., BUCHANAN, J. M.: Specific binding of azaserine with an enzyme of purine biosynthesis. Abst., 135th Meeting Amer. Chem. Soc., Boston, Mass., pp. 45—46 C. (1959).

HILF, R.: The mechanism of action of ACTH. New England J. Med. 273, 798 (1965).

HILL, J. M., ROBERTS, J., LOEB, E., KHAN, A., MACLELLAN, A., HILL, R. W.: L-Asparaginase therapy for leukaemia and other malignant lymphomas. J. Amer. med. Ass. 202, 882 (1967).

HILLEMANN, M. R.: Interferon induction and utilisation. J. cell. Physiol. 71, 43 (1968).

HIRSCHBERG, E.: Patterns of response of animal tumours to anticancer agents. Cancer Chemotherapy Screening Data. XXI. Cancer Res. 23, 521 (1963).

HITCHINGS, G. H., ELION, G. B.: Chemical suppression of the immune response. Pharmacol. Rev. 15, 365 (1963).

HO, M.: Role of infection in viral interference. I. Inhibition of lethal infections in chick embryos preinfected with influenza virus. Arch. intern. Med. 110, 653 (1962).

— Effect of an interferon on synthesis of viral ribonucleic acid and plaque formation. Proc. Soc. exp. Biol. (N. Y.) 112, 511 (1963).

— Identification and induction of interferon. Bact. Rev. 28, 367 (1964 a).

— Interferon-like viral inhibition in rabbits after intravenous administration of endotoxin. Science 146, 1472 (1964 b).

— The production of interferons. In: Interferons. Ed.: N. B. FINTER. Amsterdam: North-Holland Publishing Co. 1966, pp. 21—54.

—, BREINIG, M. K.: Conditions for the production of an interferon appearing in chick cultures infected with Sindbis virus. J. Immunol. 89, 177 (1962).

—, ENDERS, J. F.: An inhibitor of viral activity appearing in infected cell cultures. Proc. nat. Acad. Sci. (U. S.) 45, 385 (1959 a).

— — Further studies on an inhibitor of viral activity appearing in infected cell cultures and its role in chronic virus infections. Virology 9, 446 (1959 b).

—, KONO, Y.: Effect of actinomycin D on virus and endotoxin-induced interferon-like inhibitors in rabbits. Proc. nat. Acad. Sci. (U. S.) 53, 220 (1965).

—, POSTIC, B., KE, Y. H.: The systematic induction of interferon. In: Ciba Foundation Symposium on Interferons. London: Churchill 1968, p. 19.

HOFFMAN, C. E., NEUMAYER, E. M., HAFF, R. F., GOLDSBY, R. A.: Action of the antiviral activity of amantadine in tissue culture. J. Bact. 90, 623 (1965).

HOLTON, CHARLENE, VIETTI, TERESA: Remission induction of childhood leukaemia with daunomycin and prednisone. Proc. Amer. Assoc. Cancer Res. 9, 32 (1968) (Abst. 124).

HONIG, G. R., RABINOVITZ, M.: Selective suppression of nuclear-histone synthesis by actinomycin D. Fed. Proc. 23, Pt. 1, 268 (1964).

HOOK, E. W., WAGNER, R. R.: The resistance-promoting activity of endotoxins and other microbial products. II. Protection against the neurotoxic action of influenza virus. J. Immunol. 83, 310 (1959).

HOORN, B., TYRRELL, D. A.: On the growth of certain "newer" respiratory viruses in organ cultures. Brit. J. exp. Path. 46, 109 (1965).

Hori, M., Ito, E., Takita, T., Koyama, G., Takeuchi, T., Umezawa, H.: A new antibiotic, Formycin. J. Antibiot. (Tokyo) A. **17**, 96 (1964).

Horsfall, F. L., Jr., McCarty, M.: The modifying effects of certain substances of bacterial origin on the course of infection with pneumonia virus of mice (PVM). J. exp. Med. **85**, 623 (1947).

Horvath, A., de Alvarado, F., Szöcs, J., de Alvarado, Zoila N., Padilla, G.: Metabolic effects of calagualine, an antitumoural saponine of Polypodium leucotomos. Nature (Lond.) **214**, 1256 (1967).

Hosley, H. F., Marangoudakis, S., Ross, C. A., Murphy, W. T., Holland, J. F.: Combined radiation-chemotherapy for bronchogenic carcinoma—pilot study. Cancer Chemother. Rep. **16**, 467 (1962).

Huebner, R. J., Rowe, W. P., Lane, W. T.: Oncogenic effects in hamsters of human adenovirus types 12 and 18. Proc. nat. Acad. Sci. (U. S.) **48**, 2051 (1962).

Hughes, L. E.: Treatment of malignant disease with protamine sulphate. Lancet **1**, 408 (1964).

Humphrey, E. W., Blank, N.: Clinical experience with streptonigrin. Cancer Chemother. Rep. **12**, 99 (1961).

—, Dietrich, F. S.: Clinical experience with the methyl ester of streptonigrin (NCS-45384). Cancer Chemother. Rep. **33**, 21 (1963).

Hurwitz, J., Furth, J. J., Malamy, M., Alexander, M.: The role of deoxyribonucleic acid in ribonucleic acid synthesis. III. The inhibition of the enzymatic synthesis of ribonucleic acid and deoxyribonucleic acid by actinomycin D and proflavin. Proc. nat. Acad. Sci. (U. S.) **48**, 1222 (1962).

Hutchison, D. J.: Cross resistance and collateral sensitivity studies in cancer chemotherapy. Advanc. Cancer Res. **7**, 235 (1963).

Ikekawa, T., Uehara, N., Maeda, Yuko, Nakanishi, Miyako, Fukuoka, Fumika. Antiutmour activity of aqueous extracts of edible mushrooms. Cancer Res. **29**, 734 (1969).

Isaacs, A.: Mechanisms of virus infections. Nature (Lond.) **192**, 1247 (1961).

— Interferon. Advanc. Virus. Res.**10**, 1 (1963).

—, Lindenmann, J.: Proc. roy. Soc. Ser. B. **147**, 258 (1957).

Ishihara, M.: Clinical and experimental studies on chromomycin as a chemotherapeutic agent for malignant tumours. Clin. Gynecol. Obstet (Tokyo) **15**, 413 (1961). (Excerpta Med., 1962, Sect. XVI, 10, Abst. No. 4201.)

Iyer, V. N., Szybalski, W.: A molecular mechanism of mitomycin action: linking of complementary DNA strands. Proc. nat. Acad. Sci. (U. S.) **50**, 355 (1963).

— — Mitomycins and porfiromycin: chemical mechanism of activation and cross-linking of DNA. Science **145**, 55 (1964).

Jackson, L., Kofman, S., Weiss, A., Brodovsky, H.: Aristolochic acid (NSC-50413): Phase I clinical study. Cancer Chemother. Rep. **42**, 35 (1964).

Jacquillat, C., Tanger, J., Boiron, M., Najeau, Y., Weil, M., Bernard, J.: Rubidomycin. A new agent active in the treatment of acute lymphoblastic leukaemia. Lancet **1966 II**, 27.

Jensen, K. E., Neal, A. L., Owens, R. E., Warren, J.: Interferon responses of chick embryo fibroblasts to nucleic acids and related compounds. Nature (Lond.) **200**, 433 (1963).

Johnson, F., Starkovsky, N. A., Paton, A. C., Carlson, A. A.: Glutarimide antibiotics. IV. The total synthesis of dl- and l-cycloheximide. J. Amer. Chem. Soc. **86**, 118 (1964).

Johnson, I. S.: Observations on antiviral screening. Ann. N. Y. Acad. Sci. **130**, 52 (1965).

Joklik, W. K.: Studies on the mechanism of action of interferon. In: Ciba Foundation Symposium on Interferons. London: Churchill 1968, p. 110.

Journey, L. J., Goldstein, M. N.: Electron microscope studies on HeLa cells lines sensitive and resistant to actinomycin D. Cancer Res. **21**, 929 (1961).

Judge, J. W.: Inhibition of effects of leukaemogenic viruses in mice by extracts of Mercenaria mercenaria. Proc. Soc. exp. Biol. (N. Y.) **123**, 299 (1966).

Kaczka, E. A., Gitterman, C. O., Dulaney, E. L., Folkers, K.: Hadacidin, a new growth-inhibitory substance in human tumour systems. Biochemistry **1**, 340 (1962).

Kajiwara, K., Kim, U. H., Mueller, G. C.: Phleomycin, an inhibitor of replication of HeLa cells. Cancer Res. **26**, 233 (1966).

Karnofsky, D. A., Clarkson, B. D.: Cellular effects of anticancer drugs. Ann. Rev. Pharmacol. **3**, 357 (1963).

KARNOFSKY, D. A., GOLBEY, R. B., LI, M. C.: Remissions induced in trophoblastic tumours by 6-diazo-5-oxo-L-norleucine (DON). Proc. Amer. Ass. Cancer Res. 5, 33 (1964), Abst. 130.

KARON, M. R.: The role of vincristine in the treatment of childhood leukaemia. Clin. Pharmacol. Therap. 7, 332 (1966).

—, FREIREICH, E. J., FREI, E. III: A preliminary report on vincristine sulphate—a new active agent for the treatment of acute leukaemia. Pediatrics 30, 791 (1962).

KARRER, K., HUMPHREYS, S. R., GOLDIN, A.: An experimental model for studying factors which influence metastasis of malignant tumours. Int. J. Cancer 2, 213 (1967).

KATHAN, R. H.: Kelp extracts as antiviral substances. Ann. N. Y. Acad. Sci. 130, 390 (1965).

KAVERZNEVA, M. M.: Treatment of leukaemia by antitumour antibiotics olivomycin (16749) and 6613. Fed. Proc. 23, Pt. II, T. 491 (1964).

KE, Y. H., SINGER, S. H., POSTIC, B., HO, M.: Effect of puromycin on virus and endotoxin-induced interferon-like inhibitors in rabbits. Proc. Soc. exp. Biol. (N. Y.) 121, 181 (1966).

KEIDAN, S. E.: Actinomycin D in the treatment of cancer in children. Brit J. Surg. 53, 614 (1966).

KENIS, Y., STRYCKMANS, P., LEBRUN, J.: Clinical trial with mitomycin C in patients with solid tumours. In: Chemotherapy of Cancer. Ed.: A. PLATTNER. Amsterdam: Elsevier 1964, p. 153.

KENNEDY, B. J., SANDBERG-WOLLHEIM, MAGNHILD, LOKEN, MERLE, YARBRO, J. W.: Studies with tritiated mithramycin in C3H mice. Cancer Res. 27, 1534 (1967).

—, YARBRO, J. W., KECKERTZ, VIRGINIA, SANDBERG-WOLLHEIM, MAGNHILD: Effect of Mithramycin on a mouse glioma. Cancer Res. 28, 91 (1968).

KERSTEN, H., KERSTEN, W.: Die Bindung von Daunomycin, Cinerubin und Chromomycin A3 an Nukleinsäuren. Biochem. Z. 341, 174 (1965).

KERSTEN, W., KERSTEN, H., STEINER, F. E., EMMERICH, B.: Effects of chromomycin and mithramycin on the synthesis of deoxyribonucleic acid and ribonucleic acid. Hoppe-Seylers Z. physiol. Chem. 348, 1415 (1967).

KHOOBYARIAN, N., FISCHINGER, P. J.: Role of heated adenovirus 2 in viral interference. Proc. Soc. exp. Biol. (N. Y.) 120, 533 (1965).

KIDD, J. G.: Regression of transplanted lymphomas induced in vivo by means of normal guinea pig serum. I. Course of transplanted cancers of various kinds in mice and rats given guinea pig serum, horse serum or rabbit serum. J. exp. Med. 98, 565 (1953).

KIT, S., DUBBS, D. R., PIEKARSKI, L. J.: Inhibitory effects of puromycin and fluorophenyl-alanine on induction of thymidine kinase by vaccinia-infected L-cells. Biochem. Biophys. Res. Commun. 11, 176 (1963).

KLEINSCHMIDT, W. J., CLINE, J. C., MURPHY, E. B.: The production of interferon by statolon. Fed. Proc. 23, 507 (1964 a).

— — — Interferon production induced by statolon. Proc. nat. Acad. Sci. (U. S.) 52, 741 (1964 b).

—, ELLIS, L. F., VAN FRANK, R. M., MURPHY, E. B.: Interferon stimulation by a double-stranded RNA of a mycophage in statolon preparations. Nature (Lond.) 220, 167 (1968).

—, MURPHY, E. B.: Investigation on interferon induced by statolon. Virology 27, 484 (1965).

— — Interferon induction with statolon in the intact animal. Bact. Rev. 31, 132 (1967).

—, PROBST, G. W.: The nature of statolon, an antiviral agent. Antibiot. Chemother. 12, 298 (1962).

KNOCK, F. E.: Anticancer agents. Publ. C. C. Thomas, Springfield, Illinois, 1967.

KOFMAN, S., EISENSTEIN, R.: Mithramycin in the treatment of disseminated cancer. Cancer Chemother. Rep. 32, 77.

—, MEDREK, T. J., ALEXANDER, R. W.: Mithramycin in the treatment of embryonal cancer. Cancer 17, 938 (1964).

KOONS, C. R., SENSENBRENNER, L. L., OWENS, A. H., JR.: Clinical studies of mithramycin in patients with embryonal cancer. Bull. John Hopk. Hosp. 118, 462 (1966).

KORMAN, J.: Anthramycin. Cited in World Medicine, 15th August, 1967.

KORMAN, S., TENDLER, M. D.: Clinical evaluation of antibiotic Roche 5-9000. Proc. Amer. Ass. Cancer Res. 6, 37.

KORST, D. R., NIXON, J. C.: Oral administration of vinblastine sulphate (NSC-49842) to cancer patients. Cancer Chemother. Rep. 45, 53 (1965).

KUCERA, L. S., COHEN, R. A., HERRMANN, E. C., JR.: Antiviral activities of extracts of the lemon balm plant. Ann. N. Y. Acad. Sci. 130, 474 (1965).

—, HERRMANN, E. C., JR.: Gradient plate technique applied to the study of antiviral substances. Proc. Soc. exp. Biol. (N. Y.) 122, 258 (1966).

—, HERRMANN, E. C.: Antiviral substances in plants of the mint family. I. Tannin of Melissa officinalis. II. Non-tannin polyphenol of Melissa officinalis. III. Peppermint (Mentha piperita) and other mint plants. Proc. Soc. exp. Biol. (N. Y.) 124, 865—869 (1967).

KÜCHLER, C., KÜCHLER, W.: Studies of the antiviral activity of virothricin. Acta virol. (Praha) 10, 195 (1966).

KUMAGAI, K.: Antitumour activity of carzinostatin. Studies on the antibiotic substances from actinomycetes. XLV. J. Antibiot. (Tokyo) A. 15, 53 (1962).

KUPCHAN, S. M., DOSKOTCH, R. W., BOLLINGER, P., McPHAIL, A. T., SIM, G. A., SAENZ RENAULD, J. A.: The isolation and structural elucidation of a novel steroidal tumour inhibitor from Acnistus arborescens. J. Amer. Chem. Soc. 87, 5805 (1965).

—, GRAY, A. H., GROVE, M. D.: Tumour inhibitors. XXIII. The cytotoxic principles of Marah Oreganus H. J. med. Chem. 10, 337 (1967).

—, PATEL, A. C., FUJITA, E.: Tumour inhibitors. VI. Cissampareine, new cytotoxic alkaloid from Cissampelos pareira. Cytotoxicity of bisbenzylisoquinoline alkaloids. J. Pharm. Sci. 54, 580 (1965).

KURITA, S., TAKEUCHI, K., HOSHINO, A., OTO, K., KIMURA, K.: Experimental and clinical studies on resistance to mitomycin C. Gann 50, Suppl. 17 (1959).

KURODA, Y., FURUYAMA, J.: Physiological and biochemical studies of effects of mitomycin C on strain HeLa cells in cell culture. Cancer Res. 23, 682 (1963).

KURU, M.: Clinical experience with a new antitumour agent, chromomycin. Cancer Chemother. Rep. 13, 91 (1961).

KUTCHKAREV, R. N.: Olivomycin: preliminary results of clinical trials. Fed. Proc. 22, Pt. II, T. 1253 (1963).

LACHER, M. J., DURANT, J. R.: Combined vinblastine and chlorambucil therapy of Hodgkin's disease. Ann. internal Med. 62, 468 (1965).

LAMPSON, G. P., TYTELL, A. A., FIELD, A. K., NEMES, M. M., HILLEMAN, M. R.: Inducers of interferon and host resistance. I. Double-stranded RNA from extracts of Penicillium funiculosum. Proc. nat. Acad. Sci. (U. S.) 58, 782 (1967).

— —, NEMES, M. M., HILLEMAN, M. R.: Purification and characterisation of chick embryo interferon. Proc. Soc. exp. Biol. (N. Y.) 112, 468 (1963).

— — — — Characterisation of chick embryo interferon induced by a DNA virus. Proc. Soc. exp. Biol. (N. Y.) 118, 441 (1965).

LANDQUIST, J. K.: Some degradation products of fumagillin. J. Chem. Soc. 4, 4237 (1956).

LAPIS, K., BERNHARD, W.: The effect of mitomycin C on the nucleolar fine structure of KB cells in cell culture. Cancer Res. 25, 628 (1965).

LARSEN, V., MOGENSEN, B., AMRIS, C. J., STORM, O.: Fibrinolytic enzyme in the treatment of patients with cancer. Danish Med. Bull. 11, 137 (1964).

LARSON, L. M., RAUPH, W. G., HILLEMAN, M. R.: Prevention of SV40 virus tumourigenesis in newborn hamsters by maternal immunisation. Proc. Soc. exp. Biol. (N. Y.) 126, 674 (1966).

LASSMAN, L. P., PEARCE, G. W., GANG, J.: Sensitivity of intracranial gliomas to vincristine sulphate. Lancet 1965 I, 296.

— — — Effect of vincristine sulphate on the intracranial gliomata of childhood. Brit. J. Surg. 53, 774 (1966).

LEACH, B. E., FORD, J. H., WHIFFEN, A. J.: Actidione, an antibiotic from Streptomyces griseus. J. Amer. Chem. Soc. 69, 474 (1947).

LE CLERC, J. L., COGNEAUX-LE CLERC, J.: The production of interferon by two inactivated arboviruses. Acta Virol. (Praha) 9, 18 (1965).

LEHEL, F., HADHAZY, G.: Effect of heparin on herpes simplex virus infection in the rabbit. Acta microbiol. Acad. Sci. hung. 13, 197 (1966).

LEIMGRUBER, W., BATCHO, A. D., SCHENKER, F.: The structure of anthramycin. J. Amer. Chem. Soc. 87, 5793 (1965).

—, STEFANOVIC, V., SCHENKER, F., KARR, A., BERGER, J.: Isolation and characterisation of anthramycin, a new tumour antibiotic. J. Amer. Chem. Soc. 87, 5791 (1965).

LEIN, J., HEINEMANN, B., GOUREVITCH, A.: Induction of lysogenic bacteria as a method of detecting potential antitumour agents. Nature (Lond.) 196, 783 (1962).

LEMONDE, P., CLODE-HYDE, MARGARIDA: Influence of Bacille Calmette-Guérin infection on polyoma in hamsters and mice. Cancer Res. 26, 585 (1966).

LERMAN, M. I., BENYUMOVICH, M. S.: Effect of mitomycin C on protein synthesis in human neoplastic cell lines. Nature (Lond.) 206, 1231 (1965).

LESSNER, H., JONSSON, U., LOEB, V., LARSON, W.: Preliminary clinical experience with tri-methylcholchicinic acid methyl ether d-tartrate (TMCA) in various malignancies. Cancer Chemother. Rep. 27, 33 (1963).

LEVENBERG, B., MELNICK, I., BUCHANAN, J. B.: Biosynthesis of purines. XV. The effect of aza-L-serine and 6-diazo-5-oxo-L-norleucine in inosinic acid biosynthesis de novo. J. biol. Chem. 225, 163 (1957).

LEVY, H. B., BUCKLER, C. E., BARSON, S.: Effect of interferon on early interferon production. Science 152, 1274 (1966).

—, CARTER, W. A.: The mechanisms of action of interferon. In: Interferons. Ed.: N. B. FINTER. Amsterdam: North-Holland Publishing Co. 1966, pp. 160—178.

—, LAW, L. W., RABSON, A. S.: Inhibition of tumour growth by polyinosinic: polycytidylic acid. Proc. nat. Acad. Sci. (U. S.) 62, 357 (1969).

LEWIS, U. J., RICKES, E. L., McCLELLAND, LAURELLA, BRINK, N. G.: Purification and characterisation of the antiviral agent Helenine. J. Amer. Chem. Soc. 81, 4115 (1959).

LI, C. P., PRESCOTT, B., CHI, L. L., MARTINO, E. C.: Antiviral and antibacterial activity of thymus extracts. Proc. Soc. exp. Biol. (N. Y.) 114, 502 (1963).

— —, EDDY, B., CALDES, G., GREEN, W. R., MARTINO, E. C., YOUNG, A. M.: Antiviral activity of paolins from clams. Ann. N. Y. Acad. Sci. 130, 374 (1965).

— —, MARTINO, E. C., LIU, O. C.: Antineoplastic activity of clam liver extract. Nature (Lond.) 219, 1163 (1968).

LI, M. C., WHITMORE, W. F., GOLBEY, R., GRABSTALD, H.: Effects of combined drug therapy on metastatic cancer of the testis. J. Amer. med. Ass. 174, 1291 (1960).

LIKAR, M., BARTLEY, E. O., WILSON, D. C.: Observations on the interaction of poliovirus and host cells in vitro. III. The effect of some bacterial metabolites and endotoxins. Brit. J. exp. Pathol. 40, 391 (1959).

LINDENMANN, J., KLEIN, P. A.: RRCR, Vol. 9: Immunological aspects of viral oncolysis. Berlin-Heidelberg-New York: Springer 1967.

LINK, F., RADA, B., BLASKOVIC, D.: Problems of in vitro and in vivo testing of antiviral substances. Ann. N. Y. Acad. Sci. 130, 31 (1965).

LIPSETT, M. N., WEISSBACH, A.: The site of alkylation of nucleic acids by mitomycin. Biochemistry 4, 206 (1965).

LITMAN, M. L., KIM, Y. C., SUK, D.: Immunisation of mice to sarcoma 180 and Ehrlich carcinoma with ultraviolet-killed tumour vaccine. Proc. Soc. exp. Biol. (N. Y.) 127, 7 (1968).

LOCKHART, R. Z., JR.: Production of an interferon by L-cells infected with Western equine encephalomyelitis virus. J. Bact. 85, 556 (1963).

— Biological properties of interferon: criteria for acceptance of a viral inhibitor as an interferon. In: Interferons. Ed.: N. B. FINTER. Amsterdam: North-Holland Publishing Co. 1966, pp. 1—20.

LOH, P. C., CROWLEY, J. R.: Reovirus type-2 infection, cycloheximide and cell death. Proc. Soc. exp. Biol. (N. Y.) 125, 1287 (1968).

LUMB, M., MACEY, P. E., SPYVEE, J., WHITMARSH, J. M., WRIGHT, R. D.: Isolation of vivomycin and borrelidin, two antibiotics with antiviral activity from a species of Streptomyces. Nature (Lond.) 206, 263 (1965).

LUTTON, A.: Treatment of malignant disease with protamine sulphate. Lancet 1, 768 (1964).

McBRIDE, T. J., OLESON, J. J., WOOLF, D.: The activity of Streptonigrin against the Rauscher murine leukaemia virus in vivo. Cancer Res. 26, 727 (1968).

McCOWEN, M. C., CALLENDER, M. E., LAWLIS, J. F., JR.: Fumagillin (H-3) a new antibiotic with amoebicidal properties. Science 113, 202.

McCOY, J. R.: Chemotherapy of canine cancer with dihydro E-73. Fed. Proc. 19, 396 (1960).

McCRACKEN, S., ABOODY, A.: Continuous intravenous infusion of Streptonigrin (NSC-45383) in patients with bronchogenic carcinoma. Cancer Chemother. Rep. 46, 23 (1965).

McGee, A. R.: Apparent antagonism of vaccinia and wart viruses. Preliminary report on virus to virus in the tumour battle. Cancer 19, 1647 (1966).

Mackenzie, A. R.: Chemotherapy of metastatic testis cancer. Cancer 19, 1369 (1966).

Maeda, K., Kosaka, H., Yagihita, K., Umezawa, H.: A new antibiotic, phleomycin. J. Antibiot. (Tokyo) A. 9, 82 (1956).

Maevskii, M. M., Romanenko, E. A., Urazova, A. P., Molikov, Y. N., Timofeevskaya, E. A., Bondareva, A. S., Mazaeva, V. G., Talyzina, V. A., Vyazova, O. I.: Effect of olivomycin on transplanting tumours. Fed. Proc. 22, Pt. II, T. 1236 (1963).

Malpas, J. S., Scott, R. B.: Rubidomycin in acute leukaemia in adults. Brit. med. J. 3, 227 (1968).

Malucci, L.: Mouse hepatitis virus and interferon production in normal regenerating liver. Arch. ges. Virusforsch. 15, 91 (1964).

Manheimer, L. H., Vital, J.: Mitomycin C in the therapy of far-advanced malignant tumours. Cancer 19, 207 (1966).

Marsh, W. S., Garretson, A. L., Farrel, A.: E-73: an antitumour agent. Fed. Proc. 19, 305 (1960).

Mashburn, Louise T., Boyse, E. A., Campbell, H. A., Old, L. J.: A comparison of concurrent and delayed tests for antitumour activity of L-asparaginase. Proc. Soc. exp. Biol. (N. Y.) 124, 568 (1967).

—, Wriston, J. C., Jr.: Tumour inhibitory effect of L-asparaginase from Escherichia coli. Arch. Biochem. Biophys. 105, 450 (1964).

— — The change in alkaline ribonuclease levels in L-asparaginase-treated lymphosarcomas. Fed. Proc. 24, 597 (Abst. 2577) (1965).

—, Wriston, J. C.: Change in ribonuclease concentrated in L-asparaginase treated lymphosarcomata. Nature 211, 1403 (1966).

Mathé, G., Hayat, M., Schwarzenberg, L., Anniel, J. L., Schneider, M., Cattan, A., Schlumberger, J. R., Jasmin, C.: Acute lymphoblastic leukaemia treated with a combination of prednisone, vincristine, and rubidomycin. Value of pathogen-free rooms. Lancet 1967 II, 380.

Matossian, A. M., Garabedian, G. A.: Virucidal action of seawater. Amer. J. Epidemiol. 85, 1 (1967).

Matsumae, A., Yoshioka, M., Sotomura, M., Owada, H., Hata, T., Arai, H.: Experimental treatment in animals with mitomycins (1). Japan J. Microbiol. 1, 183 (1957).

Mayevsky, M. M., Kutcharev, R. N., Romanenko, E. A., Urasova, A. P., Molkov, Y. N., Timofeyevskaya, E. A., Bondareva, A. S., Masayeva, V. G., Talysina, V. A., Vyasova, O. I.: Tumour-inhibiting action of olivomycin (16749) and antibiotic 2703 "Chrysomallin". Acta Unio internat. contra Cancrum 20, 286 (1964).

Meek, E. S., Meek, Miyoko: Differential inhibition of DNA synthesis in vaccinia-infected cells by phagicin. Nature (Lond.) 220, 822 (1968).

Merigan, T. C.: Induction of circulating interferon by synthetic anionic polymers of known composition. Nature (Lond.) 214, 416 (1967 a).

— Various molecular species of interferon induced by viral and non-viral agents. Bact. Rev. 31, 138 (1967 b).

— Interferon's promise in clinical medicine. Fact or fancy? Amer. J. Med. 43, 817 (1967 c).

—, Winget, C. A., Dixon, C. B.: Purification and characterisation of vertebrate interferons. J. mol. Biol. 13, 679 (1965).

Merker, P. C., Bowie, M., Anido, P.: Effect of mithramycin and other antibiotics on a human epidermoid carcinoma growing in newborn Swiss mice. Antimicrobial Agents Chemotherapy 1961 a, pp. 148—158.

—, Pearce, F. K., Sarino, J. S., Wooley, G. W.: The effect of streptonigin and other antibiotics on a human epidermoid carcinoma, Hep/3, growing in conditioned Swiss mice. Antibiot. Chemotherap. 11, 184 (1961 b).

—, Reyes, C., Anido, P. A.: Mitomycin C-resistant Jensen rat sarcoma; isolation and transplantation studies. Cancer Res. 22, 1163.

Miller, A. J., Kimsey, Letitia S.: Biological inhibition of transplantable mouse tumours. Cancer 20, 471 (1967).

Miller, D. S., Laszlo, J., McCarty, K. S., Guild, W. R., Hochstein, P.: Mechanism of action of streptonigrin in leukaemic cells. Cancer Res. 27, 632 (1967).

MILLER, E., SULLIVAN, R. D., CHRYSSOCHOOS, T.: The clinical effects of mitomycin C by continuous intravenous administration. Cancer Chemother. Rep. 21, 129 (1962).

MILLER, F. A., RIGHTSEL, W. A., SLOAN, B. J., EHRLICH, J., FRENCH, J. C., BARTZ, Q. R., DIXON, G. J.: Antiviral activity of tenuazonic acid. Nature (Lond.) 200, 1338 (1963).

—, WHEELOCK, DIANE: Assaying of antiviral activity of tenuazonic acid in cell culture. In: Antimicrobial Agents and Chemotherapy. Ed.: GLADYS L. HOBBY. 1965, pp. 360—363.

MILLER, P. A., MILSTREY, K. P., TROWN, P. W.: Specific inhibition of viral ribonucleic acid replication by gliotoxin. Science 159, 431 (1968).

MIRO-QUESADA, O., AYULO, V. M., ADACHI, L.: Experimental combination treatment of disseminated cancer in man with mitomycin C, "Ayulo's Filtrate", prednisolone and/or androgen. Cancer Chemother. Rep. 13, 113 (1961).

MIYAMURA, S.: A determination method for anticancer action of antibiotics by the agar plate diffusion technique. Antibiot. Chemother. 6, 280 (1956).

—, NIWAYAMA, S.: An agar diffusion method using HeLa cells for antitumour screening. Antibiot. Chemother. 9, 497 (1959).

MIYAZAKI, K., TSUNODA, A., RIKIMARU, M., ISHIDA, N.: On the chemoprophylactic effect of miromycin against poliovirus infection. J. Antibiot. (Tokyo) A. 16, 51 (1963).

MOHR, U., ALTHOFF, J., KINZEL, V., SÜSS, R., VOLM, M.: Melanoma regression induced by "Chalone": a new tumour inhibiting principle acting in vivo. Nature (Lond.) 220, 138 (1968).

MONOD, J., CHANGEUX, J. P., JACOB, F.: Allosteric proteins and cellular control systems. J. mol. Biol. 6, 306 (1963).

MOORE, A. E.: Viruses with oncolytic properties and their adaptation to tumours. Ann. N. Y. Acad. Sci. 54, 945 (1952).

— The oncolytic viruses. Progr. exp. Tumour Res. 1, 411 (1960).

MÖSE, J. R., MÖSE, G.: Oncolysis by Clostridia. I. Activity of Clostridium butyricum (M-55) and other nonpathogenic Clostridia against the Ehrlich carcinoma. Cancer Res. 24, 212 (1964).

MOUNTAIN, ISABEL M., CAPPUCINO, J. G., MUELLER, C. M., RITTER, F. W., SCHMID, F. A., SMOL, BARBARA A., TARNOWSKI, G. S.: Chemotherapy studies in an animal tumour spectrum. III. Evaluation of the toxicity differential index. Cancer Res. 26, 258 (1966).

MURATA, T., ARAKAWA, M., SUGIYA, Y., INAZU, Y., HATTORI, Z., SUZUKI, Y., MINAKAMI, H., NAKAHARA, M., OKAZAKI, H.: Oncolytic effect of Proteus mirabilis upon tumour-bearing animal. Life Sci. 4, 1055 (1965).

MURRAY-LYON, I. M., EDDLESTON, A. L. W. F., WILLIAMS, R., BROWN, M., HOGBIN, B. M., BENNET, A., EDWARDS, J. C., TAYLOR, K. W.: Treatment of multiple-hormone-producing malignant islet-cell tumour with streptozotocin. Lancet 2, 895 (1968).

MURTHY, Y. K. S., THIEMANN, J. E., CORONELLI, C., SENSI, P.: Alanosine, a new antiviral and antitumour agent isolated from a streptomyces. Nature (Lond.) 211, 1198 (1966).

MYLES, A. B.: A trial of vinblastine sulphate in the treatment of inoperable carcinoma of the lung. Brit. J. Cancer 20, 264 (1966).

NAFICY, K., CARVER, D. H.: "Cyclopin"; a trypsin sensitive constituent of Penicillium cyclopium with antiviral properties. Proc. Soc. exp. Biol. (N. Y.) 114, 175 (1963).

NAGANO, Y., KOHIMA, Y.: Inhibition de l'infection vaccinale par un facteur liquide dans le tissu infecte par le virus homologue. Compt. rend. Soc. Biol. 152, 1627 (1958).

NAKAHARA, W., FUKUOKA, F., MAEDA, Y., AOKI, K.: The host-mediated antitumour effect of some plant polysaccharides. Gann 55, 283 (1964).

— —, SUGIMURA, T., HOZUMI, M.: Ein carcinostatischer Leber-Faktor. Naturwissenschaften 50, 406 (1963).

NAKAZAWA, M., KASAI, N., YAMAMOTO, T.: Studies on carcinostatic activity of phosphomucolipid (PML) obtained from liposaccharide. Proc. Ninth internat. Cancer Congress, Tokyo, 1966, p. 334, Abst. S. 0582 (1966).

NATHANS, D., NEIDLE, A.: Structural requirements for puromycin inhibition of protein synthesis. Nature (Lond.) 197, 1076 (1963).

NELSON, J. B., TARNOWSKY, G. S.: An oncolytic virus recovered from Swiss mice during passage of an ascites tumour. Nature (Lond.) 188, 866 (1960).

NEUSS, N., GORMAN, M., JOHNSON, I. S.: Natural products in cancer chemotherapy. In: Methods in Cancer Research. Ed.: H. BUSCH. London: Academic Press 1967, Vol. III, pp. 633.

NIGRELLI, R. F., JAKOWSKA, S.: Effects of holothurin, a steroid saponin from the Bahamian sea cucumber (Actinopyga agassizi) on various biological systems. Ann. N. Y. Acad. Sci. 90, 884 (1960).

NISHIYAMA, S., KATAGIRI, K.: Antiviral activity of minomycin against poliomyelitis in mice. Ann. Rept. Shionogi Res. Lab. 210 (1964).

NISHMI, M.: Effect of "Cephaloridine" on vaccinia virus in vitro. Nature (Lond.) 209, 222 (1966).

NOBLE, R. L., BEER, C. T., CUTTS, J. H.: Role of chance observations in chemotherapy: Vinca rosea. Ann. N. Y. Acad. Sci. 76, 882 (1958).

OBOSHI, S.: Cross-resistance between mitomycin C and alkylating agents in experimental cancer chemotherapy. Gann 50, 147 (1959).

ODA, M.: Vaccinia virus—HeLa cell interaction. II. The effect of mitomycin C in the production of infective virus, complement-fixing antigen, and haemagglutinin. Virology 21, 533 (1963).

OETTGEN, H. F., OLD, L. J., BOYSE, E. A., CAMPBELL, H. A., PHILLIPS, F. S., CLARKSON, B. D., TALLAL, L., LEEPER, R. D., SCHWARTZ, M. K., KIM, J. H.: Inhibition of leukaemias in man by L-asparaginase. Cancer Res. 27, 2619 (1967).

OH, J. O.: An interferon-like viral inhibitor in body fluids of endotoxin-injected rabbits. Proc. Soc. exp. Biol. (N. Y.) 123, 493 (1966).

OHNO, S., NOZIMA, T.: Inhibitory effect of interferon on the induction of thymidine kinase in vaccinia virus-infected chick embryo fibroblasts. Acta Virol. (Praha) 8, 479 (1964).

OKAMOTO, H.: Report to Japan Pharmacological Society, cited in World Medicine, 12th July 1968, p. 35.

OLD, L. J., BOYSE, E. A., CAMPBELL, H. A., BRODEY, R. S., FIDLER, J., TELLER, J. D.: Treatment of lymphosarcoma in the dog with L-asparaginase. Lancet 1, 447 (1967).

OLESON, J. J., CALDERELLA, L. A., MJOS, K. J., REITH, A. R., THIE, R. S., TOPLIN, I.: The effects of streptonigrin on experimental tumours. Antibiot. Chemother. 11, 158 (1961).

OLSON, B. H., GOERNER, G. L.: Alpha sarcin, a new antitumour agent. I. Isolation, purification, chemical composition and the identity of a new amino acid. Appl. Microbiol. 13, 314 (1965).

—, JENNINGS, J. C., ROGA, V., JUNEK, A. J., SCHUURMANS, D. M.: Alpha sarcin, a new antitumour agent. II. Fermentation and antitumour spectrum. Appl. Microbiol. 13, 322 (1965).

O'MEARA, R. A. Q., O'HALLORAN, M. J.: Protamine derivatives in the treatment of advanced carcinoma of the breast. Lancet 2, 613 (1963).

OTSUKA, H., EGYÜD, L. G.: Nucleic acid and protein synthesis of malignant ascites cells in the presence of liver extract and methyl glyoxal. Cancer Res. 27, 1498 (1967).

—, TERAYAMA, H.: Inhibition of DNA synthesis in ascites hepatoma cells by normal liver extract. Biochem. biophys. acta 123, 274 (1966).

OWEN, S. P., DIETZ, A., CAMIENER, G. W.: Sparsomycin, a new antitumour antibiotic. I. Discovery and biological properties. Antimicrobial Agents Chemotherapy (1962), pp. 772—779.

—, SMITH, C. G.: Cytotoxicity and antitumour properties of the abnormal nucleoside tubericidin (NSC-56408). Cancer Chemother. Rep. 36, 19 (1964).

OXFORD, J. S., SCHILD, G. C.: The evaluation of antiviral compounds for rubella virus using organ cultures. Arch. ges. Virusforsch. 22, 349 (1967).

PACK, G. T.: In: Progress in clinical cancer. Ed.: I. M. AIREL. New York: Grune & Stratton 1964, p. 1.

PARKER, G. W., WILTSIE, D. S., JACKSON, C. B.: The clinical evaluation of PA-144 (mithramycin) in solid tumours of adults. Cancer Chemother. Rep. 8, 23 (1960).

PARSHLEY, MARY S.: Effect of inhibitory from adult connective tissue on growth of a series of human tumours in vitro. Cancer Res. 25, 387 (1965).

PATRICK, J. B., WILLIAMS, R. P., MEYER, W. E., FULMOR, W., COSULICH, D. B., BROSCHARD, R. W., WEBB, J. S.: Aziridinomitosenes: a new class of antibiotics related to the mitomycins. J. Amer. Chem. Soc. 86, 1889 (1964).

PAUCKER, K.: The serologic specificity of interferon. J. Immunol. 94, 371 (1965).

PAUKER, K., SKURSKA, Z., HENLE, W.: Quantitative studies on viral interferences in suspended L cells. I. Growth characteristics and interfering activities of vesicular stomatitis, Newcastle disease, and influenza A viruses. Virology 17, 301 (1962).

PETTIT, G. R., HARTWELL, J. L., WOOD, H. B.: Arthropod antineoplastic agents. Cancer Res. 28, 2168 (1968).

PIAZZA, M., PANE, G., PICCIOTTO, L., LOMBARDI, D.: Effect of the infectivity of various viruses by the intestinal factor of normal mice which inactivates murine hepatitis virus. Nature (Lond.) 213, 293 (1967).

PIENTA, R. J., BERNSTEIN, E. H., GROUPÉ, V.: Experiences with virus-induced Rous sarcoma as a model in experimental therapy. Cancer Chemother. Rep. 31, 25 (1963).

PIETSCH, P.: Reactions of phleomycin and DNA. J. Cell. Biol., 31, 86 A (1966).

PILCH, Y. H., RIGGINS, R. S.: Antibodies to spontaneous and methylcholanthrene-induced tumours in mice. Cancer Res. 26, 871 (1966).

PINNERT-SINDICO, S., NINET, L., PREUD'HOMME, J., COSAR, C.: A new antibiotic: spiramycin. Antibiot. Ann. (1955), p. 724.

PLANELLES, J. J., SOLOVYEVA, Y. A., BELOVA, Z. N., SILAEV, A. B., EBERT, M. K., GRACHEVA, N. P., KHARITONOVA, A. M., GOSHEVA, A. E., AKOPYANTS, S. S.: Aurantin—a complex antibiotic substance of the actinomycin group: its properties and results of clinical trials on various types of neoplasms. Acta Unio intern. contra Cancrum 20, 297 (1964).

PONS, M.: Effect of actinomycin D on the replication of influenza virus and influenza virus RNA. Virology 33, 150 (1967).

PORTER, J. N., HEWITT, R. I., HESSELTINE, C. W., KRUPKA, G., LOWERY, J. A., WALLACE, W. S., BOHONOS, N., WILLIAMS, J. H.: Achromycin: a new antibiotic having trypanocidal properties. Chemotherapy 2, 409 (1952).

POTTER, V. R.: Biochemical perspectives in Cancer. Cancer Res. 24, 1085 (1964).

POWELL, H. M., CULBERTSON, C. G., McGUIRE, J. M., HOEHN, M. W., BAKER, L. A.: Filtrate with chemoprophylactic and chemotherapeutic action against MN and Semliki Forest viruses in mice. Antibiot. Chemotherapy 2, 432 (1952).

PRESCOTT, B., CALDES, G.: Chemical studies of an antitumour substance from clams. Fed. Proc. 26, 314 (Abst. 336) (1967).

—, LI, C. P., MARTINO, E. C., CALDES, G.: Isolation and characterisation of antiviral substance from marine animals. Fed. Proc. 23, 508 (1964).

RABINOWITZ, M., FISHER, J. M.: A dissociative effect of puromycin on the pathway of protein synthesis by Ehrlich ascites tumour cells. J. biol. Chem. 237, 477 (1962).

RADA, B., BLASKOVIC, D., SORM, F., SKODA, J.: The inhibitory effect of 6-azauracil riboside on the multiplication of vaccinia virus. Experientia 16, 487 (1960).

RAKIETEN, N., RAKIETEN, M. L., NADKARNI, M. V.: Studies on the diabetogenic action of strepozotocin (NSC-37917). Cancer Chemother. Rep. 29, 91 (1963).

RAMANATHAN, S., FURUSAWA, E., READ, G., CUTTING, W.: Isolation and activity of propionin A, and antiviral polypeptide from Propionibacteria. Chemotherapia 10, 197 (1966 a).

—, READ, G., CUTTINNG, W.: Purification of Propionin, an antiviral agent from Propionibacteria. Proc. Soc. exp. Biol. (N. Y.) 123, 271 (1966 b).

—, WOLYNEC, C., CUTTING, W.: Antiviral principles of Propionibacteria—isolation and activity of propionins B and C. Proc. Soc. exp. Biol. (N. Y.) 129, 73 (1968).

RAO, K. V.: E-73; an antitumour substance. Pt. II Structure. J. Amer. Chem. Soc. 82, 1129 (1960).

— Chemistry of duazomycins. I. Duazomycin A. Antimicrobial Agents Chemotherapy 1961, pp. 178—183.

— E-73, an antitumour substance: III. Some derivatives. Antibiot. Chemother. 12, 123 (1962).

—, BIEMANN, K., WOODWARD, R. B.: The structure of streptonigrin. J. Amer. Chem. Soc. 85, 2532 (1963).

—, BROOKS, S. C., KUGELMAN, M., ROMANO, A. A.: Diazomycins A, B and C, three antitumour substances. I. Isolation and characteristics. Antibiot. Ann. 1960, p. 943.

—, CULLEN, W. P.: E-73: an antitumour substance. Pt. I. Isolation and characterisation. J. Amer. Chem. Soc. 82, 1127 (1960 a).

— — Streptonigrin, an antitumour substance. I. Isolation and characterisation. Antibiot. Ann. 1960 b, pp. 950—953.

RAO, K. V., CULLEN, W. P., SOBIN, B. A.: Mithramycin, an antibiotic with antitumour properties. Proc. Amer. Ass. Cancer Res. 3, 143 (1960).
— — — A new antibiotic with antitumour properties. Antibiot. Chemother. 12, 182 (1962).
REEMSTSMA, K., RYAN, R. F., KREMEMTZ, E. T., CREECH, O., JR.: Treatment of selected adenocarcinomas by perfusion technique. A.M.A. Arch. Surg. 78, 727 (1959).
REICH, E.: Biochemistry of actinomycins. Cancer Res. 23, 1428 (1963).
—, FRANKLIN, R. M.: Effect of mitomycin C on the growth of some animal viruses. Proc. nat. Acad. Sci. (U. S.) 47, 1212 (1961).
—, GOLDBERG, I. H., RABINOWITZ, M.: Structure-activity correlations of actinomycins and their derivatives. Nature (Lond.) 196, 743 (1962).
REILLY, H. CHRISTINE: An evaluation of the use of antimicrobial activity as a screening procedure for tumour-inhibiting agents. Cancer Res., Suppl. 3, 63 (1955).
—, SUGIURA, K.: An antitumour spectrum of streptonigrin. Antibiot. Chemother. 11, 174 (1961).
RENIS, H. E., JOHNSON, H. G., BHUYAN, B. K.: A collagen plate assay for cytotoxic agents. I. Methods. Cancer Res. 22, 1126 (1962).
RHIM, J. A., GREENWALT, CHARLOTTE, HUEBNER, R. J.: Synthetic Double-Stranded RNA: Inhibitory effect on murine leukaemia and sarcoma viruses in cell cultures. Nature (Lond.) 222, 1166 (1969).
RICHARDS, J. F., JONES, R. G. W., BEER, C. T.: Biochemical studies with the Vinca alkaloids. I. Effects on nucleic acid formation by isolated cell suspensions. Cancer Res. 26, Pt. I, 876 (1966).
RIGHTSEL, W. A., SCHNEIDER, H. G., SLOAN, B. J., GRAF, P. R., MILLER, F. A., BARTZ, Q. R., EHRLICH, J.: Antiviral activity of gliotoxin and gliotoxin acetate. Nature (Lond.) 204, 1333 (1964).
RILEY, V.: Role of the LDH-elevating virus in leukaemia therapy by asparaginase. Nature (Lond.) 220, 1245 (1968).
RIVERS, S. L., WHITTINGTON, R. M., MEDREK, T.: Methyl ester of streptonigrin (NSC-45384) in treatment of malignant lymphoma. Cancer Chemother. Rep. 46, 17 (1965).
— — — Treatment of malignant lymphomas with methyl ester of streptonigrin (NSC-45384). Cancer 19, 1377 (1966).
ROBERTS, J., PRAGER, M. D., BACHYNSKY, N.: The antitumour activity of Escherichia coli L-asparaginase. Cancer Res. 26, 2213 (1966).
ROLAND, J. F., CHMIELEWICZ, Z. F., WEINER, B. A., GROSS, A. M., BOENING, O. P., LUCK, J. V., BARDOS, T. J., REILLY, H. CHRISTINE, SUGIURA, K., STOCK, C. C., LUCAS, E. H., BYERRUM, R. U., STEVENS, J. A.: Calvacin: a new antitumour agent. Science 132, 1897 (1960).
ROSENOER, V. M.: Methods of drug evaluation. In: Experimental Chemotherapy. Eds.: R. J. SCHNITZER and F. HAWKINS. New York: Academic Press 1966, Vol. IV, pp. 9—77.
ROSS, G. T., STOLBACH, L. L., HERTZ, R.: Actinomycin D in the treatment of methotrexate-resistant trophobastic disease in women. Cancer Res. 22, 1015 (1962).
ROSSOLIMO, O. K., LEPESHKINA, G. N.: Antitumour effect of olivomycin combined with various synthetic cytotoxic drugs. Fed. Proc. 23, Pt. II, T. 484 (1964).
ROTEM, Z., BERWALD, Y., SACHS, L.: Inhibition of interferon production in hamster cells transformed in vitro with carcinogenic hydrocarbons. Virology 24, 483 (1964).
—, COX, R. A., ISAACS, A.: Inhibition of virus multiplication by foreign nucleic acid. Nature (Lond.) 197, 564 (1963).
RUBIN, R. J., REYNARD, A., HANDSCHUMACHER, R. E.: An analysis of the lack of drug synergism during sequential blockade of de novo pyrimidine biosynthesis. Cancer Res. 24, 1002 (1964).
RYTEL, M. W., SHOPE, R. E., KILBOURNE, E. D.: An antiviral substance from Penicillium funiculosum. V. Induction of interferon by helenine. J. exp. Med. 123, 577 (1966).
RYTÖMAA, R., KIVINIEMI, KYLLIKKI: Control of cell production in rat chloroleukaemia by means of granulocytic chalone. Nature (Lond.) 220, 136 (1968).
SABIN, A. B.: Different effect of chloramphenicol, dactinomycin and streptovitacin A on synthesis of tumour and virion antigens in SV-40 virus-infected cells. Proc. nat. Acad. Sci. (U. S.) 55, 1141 (1966).

SALGANIK, R. I., MARTYNOVA, R. P., MATIENKO, N. A., RONICHEVSKAYA, G. M.: Effect on deoxyribonuclease on the course of lymphatic leukaemia in AKR mice. Nature (Lond.) 214, 100 (1967).

SAMPEY, J. R.: Alkaloids of Vinca rosea in leukaemia. Lancet 2, 392 (1966).

SARTORELLI, A. C., BOOTH, B. A.: The synergistic inhibition of sarcoma 180 by combinations of mitomycin C with either 6-thioguanine or 5-fluorouracil. Proc. Amer. Ass. Cancer Res. 5, 55 (1964).

SATHER, G. E., HAMMON, W. McD.: A tissue culture interference test for dengue viruses. Fed. Proc. 22, 557, Abst. 2370 (1963).

SCHABEL, F. M., JR., PITILLO, R. F.: Screening for and biological characterisation of anti-tumour agents using micro-organisms. Advanc. Appl. Microbiol. 3, 223 (1961).

SCHAFFER, F. L., GORDON, MARJORIE: Differential inhibitory effects of actinomycin D among strains of poliovirus. J. Bact. 91, 2309 (1966).

SCHEPARTZ, S. A., ABBOTT, B. J., LEITER, J.: Screening data from the Cancer Chemotherapy National Service Center Screening Laboratories. XLV. Cancer Res. 27, Pt. 2, 1115 (1967).

—, MacDONALD, M., LEITER, J.: The use of cell culture as a presumptive screen for anti-tumour agents. Proc. Amer. Ass. Cancer Res. 3, 265 (1961).

SCHMEER, ROSARII M.: Growth-inhibiting agents from Mercenaria extracts: chemical and biological properties. Science 144, 413 (1964).

SCHMITZ, H., BRADNER, W. T., GOUREVITCH, A., HEINEMANN, B., PRICE, K. E., LEIN, J., HOOPER, I. R.: Actinogan; a new antitumour agent obtained from Streptomyces. I. Chemical and biological properties. Cancer Res. 22, 163 (1962).

—, DE VAULT, R. L., HOOPER, I. R.: Peptinogan, a polypeptide moiety of actinogan with antitumour properties. J. med. Chem. 6, 613 (1963).

SCHNITZER, R. J.: Drug resistance in chemotherapy. In: Experimental Chemotherapy, Vol. IV. Eds.: R. J. SCHNITZER and F. HAWKING. New York: Academic Press 1966.

SCHREK, R., DOLOWY, W. C., AMMERAAL, R. N.: L-asparaginase toxicity to normal and leukaemic human lymphocytes. Science 155, 329 (1967).

SCHUURMANS, D. M., DUNCAN, D. T., OLSON, B. H.: An agar plate, assay for anticancer agents utilising serially cultured sarcoma 180 (Foley). Antibiot. Chemother. 10, 535 (1960).

— — — A bioautographic system employing mammalian cell strain and its application to antitumoral antibiotics. Cancer Res. 24, 83 (1964).

SCHWARTZ, H. S., STERNBERG, S. S., PHILIPS, F. S.: Pharmacology of mitomycin C. IV. Effects in vivo on nucleic acid synthesis; comparison with actinomycin. Cancer Res. 23, 1125 (1963).

SCOTT, W. P., VOIGHT, J. A.: Kaposi's sarcoma: management with vincaleucoblastine. Cancer 19, 557 (1966).

SEGALOFF, A.: Results of studies of the cooperative breast cancer group, 1961—1963. Cancer Chemother. Rep. 41, Suppl. 1, 1 (1964).

SETÄLÄ, K.: Further evidence for the incompatible pharmacodynamic responses to colchicine of malignant and of benign epidermal hyperplasia in mice of skin tumour-resistant strain. Naturwissenschaften 52, 520 (1965).

—, HUGANEN, A., LINDROOS, B., NYSSÖNEN, O.: Disparities in the modes of pharmacodynamic response to colchicine of malignant and of benign epidermal hyperplasia in skin-tumour-susceptible Swiss CF 1 mice. Naturwissenschaften 52, 519 (1965).

SEWELL, I. A., ELLIS, H.: A trial of mithramycin in the treatment of advanced malignant disease. Brit. J. Cancer 20, 256 (1966).

SHAH, V. C., REILLY, P.: Effect of histones, other basic proteins and some antibiotics on the transplantability of mouse mammary tumours. Nature 213, 403 (1967).

SHIGEURA, H. T., GORDON, C. N.: Hadacidin, a new inhibitor of purine biosynthesis. J. biol. Chem. 237, 1932 (1962 a).

— — The mechanism of action of hadacidin. J. biol. Chem. 237, 1937 (1962 b).

SHOHAT, B., GITTER, S., LAVIE, D.: Action of elatericin A on human leukamic and normal lymphocytes. J. nat. Cancer Inst. 38, 1 (1967).

— —, LEVIE, B., LAVIE, D.: The combined effect of cucurbitacine and X-ray treatment on transplanted tumours in mice. Cancer Res. 25, 1828 (1965).

SHOJI, J.: Preliminary studies on the isolation of carzinostatin complex and its characteristics. Studies on the Streptomyces antibiotics. XLIII. J. Antibiot. (Tokyo) A 14, 27 (1961).

SHOPE, R. E.: An antiviral substance from Penicillium funiculosum. I. Effect upon infection in mice with swine influenza virus and Columbia SK encephalomyelitis virus. J. exp. Med. 97, 601 (1953 a).
— An antiviral substance from Penicillium funiculosum. II. Effect of helenine upon infection in mice with Semliki Forest virus. J. exp. Med. 97, 627 (1953 b).
— An antiviral substance from Penicillium funiculosum. III. General properties and characteristics of helenine. J. exp. Med. 97, 639 (1953 c).
— An antiviral substance from Penicillium funiculosum. IV. Inquiry into the mechanism by which helenine exerts its antiviral effect. J. exp. Med. 123, 213 (1966).
SIMINOFF, P.: A plaque suppression method for the study of antiviral compounds. Appl. Microbiol. 9, 66 (1961).
—, HURSKY, V. S.: Determination of mammalian cell (strain HeLa) inhibition by an agar diffusion technic. I. Quantitative assay methods. Cancer Res. 20, 615 (1960).
SKIPPER, H. E.: Perspectives in cancer chemotherapy: therapeutic design. Cancer Res. 24, 1295 (1964).
—, SCHMIDT, L. H.: A manual on quantitative drug evaluation in experimental tumours systems. Pt. I. Background description of criteria and presentation of quantitative therapeutic data on various classes of drugs obtained in diverse experimental tumour systems. Cancer Chemother. Rep. 17, 1 (1962).
—, WILCOX, W. S., SCHABEL, F. M., JR., LASTER, W. R., JR., MATTIL, L.: Experimental evaluation of potential anticancer agents. X. A specificity test for distinguishing false positives. Cancer Chemother. Rep. 29, 1 (1963).
SMITH, C. G., LUMMIS, W. L., GRADY, J. E.: An improved tissue culture assay. I. Methodology and cytotoxicity of antitumour agents. Cancer Res. 19, 843 (1959 a).
— — — An improved tissue culture assay. II. Cytotoxicity studies with antibiotics, chemicals and solvents. Cancer Res. 19, 847 (1959 b).
— — — Studies on the mode of action streptovitacin A. Cancer Res. 21, 1394 (1960).
SMITH, R. D., HENSON, D., GEHRKE, J., BARTON, J. R.: Reversible inhibition of DNA virus replication with mithramycin. Proc. Soc. exp. Biol. (N. Y.) 122, 209 (1966).
SMITHERS, D.: Metabolic effects of actinobolin. Proc. Amer. Ass. Cancer Res. 7, 66, Abst. 261 (1966).
SOEDA, M.: Studies on marinamycin, an antitumour antibiotic substance. Cancer Chemother. Rep. 18, 9 (1962 a).
— Protective and chemotherapeutic effects of marinamycin against leukopenia in rabbits. Cancer Chemotherapy Abst. 4, 63, No. 1630 (1963) citing Nippon Acta Radiol. 22, 199 (1962 b).
SOKOLSKI, W. T., EILERS, N. J., SAVAGE, G. M.: Paper chromatography and microbiological assay of the streptovitacins. Antibiot. Ann. 1959, pp. 551—554.
SOLOMON, J. J., GLATT, K. A., OKAZAKI, W.: Inhibitory effect of heparin on RSV. J. Bact. 92, 1855 (1966).
SOMERSON, N. L., COOK, N. K.: Suppression of Rous sarcoma virus growth in tissue culture by Mycoplasma orale. J. Bact. 90, 534 (1965).
SONNABEND, J. A., FRIEDMAN, R. M.: Mechanism of interferon action. In: Interferons. Ed.: N. B. FINTER. Amsterdam: North-Holland Publishing Co. 1966, pp. 202—231.
—, MARTIN, E. M., MECS, E.: The effect of interferon on the synthesis and activity of an RNA polymerase isolated from chick cells infected with Semliki Forest virus. J. gen. Virol. 1, 41 (1967).
SOUTHAM, C. N.: Present status of oncolytic virus studies. Trans. N. Y. Acad. Sci., Ser. II, 22, 657 (1960).
SPEAR, P. W.: Clinical trrial with mithramycin. Cancer Chemother. Rep. 29, 109 (1963).
STÄHELIN, H., CERLETTI, A.: Experimentelle Ergebnisse mit den Podophyllum-Cytostica SP-1 und SP-G. Schweiz. med. Wochschr. 94, 1490 (1964).
STARR, T. J., DEIG, E. F., CHURCH, K., ALLEN, M. B.: Antibacterial and antivirus activities of algal extracts studied by acridine orange staining. Texas Rept. Biol. Med. 20, 271 (1962).
STEPHENS, F. O.: Evidence for a physiological antineoplastic substance in avian eggs. Lancet 1, 243 (1964).

STERNBERG, S. S., PHILIPS, F. S., CRONIN, A. P., SODERGREN, J. E., VIDAL, P. M.: Toxicological studies of calvacin. Cancer Res. 23, 1036 (1963).

STILL, R. N.: The vinca alkaloids in female genital cancer. J. Obstet. Gynaecol. Brit. Commonwealth 73, 621 (1966).

STINEBRING, W. R., YOUNGNER, J. S.: Patterns of interferon appearance in mice injected with bacteria or bacterial endotoxin. Nature (Lond.) 204, 712 (1964).

STOCK, C. C.: Preclinical studies and the characterisation of new antitumour agents. Illumination from a tumour system. Acta Unio intern. contra Cancrum 20, 41 (1964).

—, REILLY, H. C., BUCKLEY, S. M., CLARKE, D. A., RHOADS, C. P.: Azaserine, a new tumour-inhibitory substance. Studies with Crocker mouse sarcoma 180. Nature (Lond.) 173, 71 (1954).

STOCK, J. A.: Antitumour antibiotics. In: Experimental Chemotherapy, Vol. IV. Eds.: R. J. SCHNITZER and F. HAWKING. London: Academic Press 1966, pp. 239—377.

STOLINSKY, D. C., JACOBS, E. M., BATEMAN, J. R., HZEN, J. G., KUZMA, J. W., WOOD, D. A., STENFELD, J. L.: Clinical trial of trimethyl colchicine acid methyl ether d-tartrate (TMCA; NSC-36354) in advanced cancer. Cancer Chemother. Rep. 51, 25 (1967).

STONE, R. L., DE LONG, D. C., HULL, R. N., JOHNSON, I. S.: In vivo and in vitro inhibition of hepatitis virus by streptothricin. Ann. N. Y. Acad. Sci. 130, 355 (1965).

SUBAK-SHARPE, J. H., TIMBURY, M. C., WILLIAMS, J. F.: Rifampicin inhibits the growth of some mammalian viruses. Nature (Lond.) 222, 341 (1969).

SUGIURA, K.: The effect of antibiotics on a spectrum of tumours. Antibiot. Ann. 1960, pp. 924—942.

— Antitumour activity of mitomycin C. Cancer Chemother. Rep. 13, 51 (1961).

—, STOCK, C. C., REILLY, H. C., SCHMID, M. M.: Studies in a tumour spectrum. VII. The effects of antibiotics on the growth of a variety of mouse, rat and hamster tumours. Cancer Res. 18, 66 (1958).

SULLIVAN, MARGARET P., BEATTY, E. C., HYMAN, C. B., MURPHY, M. L., PIERCE, M. I., SEVERO, N. C.: A comparison of the effectiveness of standard dose 6-mercaptopurine, combination 6-mercaptopurine and DON, and high-loading 6-mercaptopurine therapies in the treatment of the acute leukaemias of childhood; results of a cooperative study. Cancer Chemother. Rep. 18, 83 (1962).

—, SUTOW, W. W., CANGIR, A., TAYLOR, G.: Vincristine sulphate in the management of Wilms' tumour. Replacement of preoperative irradiation by chemotherapy. J. Amer. med. Ass. 202, 381 (1967).

SUZUKI, S., MARUMO, S.: Chemical structure of tubericidin. J. Antibiot. (Tokyo) A. 14, 34 (1961).

SVOBODA, G. H., POORE, G. A., SIMPSON, P. J., et al.: Alkaloids of Acronychia Baueri Schott. I. Isolation of the alkaloid and a study of antitumour and other biological properties of acronycine. J. Pharm. Sci. 55, 758 (1966).

SZENT-GYÖRGYI, A.: Cell division and cancer. Science 149, 34 (1965).

—, HEGYELI, A., McLAUGHLIN, JANE A.: Constituents of the thymus gland and their relation to growth, fertility, muscle and cancer. Proc. nat. Acad. Sci. (U. S.) 48, 1439 (1962).

SZYBALSKI, W., IYER, V. N.: Crosslinking of DNA by enzymatically or chemically activated mitomycins and porfiromycins bifunctionally "alkylating" antibiotics. Fed. Proc. 23, 946 (1964).

TAKANO, K., WARREN, J., JENSEN, K. E., NEAL, A. L.: Nucleic acid-induced resistance to viral infection. J. Bact. 90, 1542 (1965).

TAKEMOTO, K. K., BARON, S.: Non-heritable interferon resistance in a fraction of virus populations. Proc. Soc. exp. Biol. (N. Y.) 121, 670 (1966).

—, LIEBHABER, N.: Virus polysaccharide interactions. I. An agar polysaccharide determining plaque morphology of EMC virus. Virology 14, 456 (1962).

TAKENAKA, Y., OGAWA, Y., ODASHIRO, T., KARUBE, N.: Anticancer activity of Gentiana extract. Ann. Rept. Nat. Inst. Genetics (Japan), No. 11, 63 (1961).

TALLAL, LISA, OETTGEN, H.: Treatment of acute leukaemia in children with L-asparaginase. Proc. Amer. Ass. Cancer Res. 9, 70 (Abst. 276) (1968).

TAN, C., TASAKA, H., DI MARCO, A.: Clinical studies of daunomycin. Proc. Amer. Ass. Cancer Res. 6, 64, Abst. 253 (1965).

TAN, C. T., DARGEON, H. W., BURCHENAL, J. H.: The effect of actinomycin D on cancer in childhood. Pediatrics 24, 544 (1959).

TAN, C. T. C., COLBEY, R. B., YAPP. C. L., WOLLNER, N., HACKETHAL, C. A., MURPHY, L. M., DARGEON, H. W., BURCHENAL, J. H.: Clinical experiences with actinomycin D, KS2 and F1 (KS4). Ann. N. Y. Acad. Sci. 9, 426 (1960).

TAN, CHARLOTTE, TASAKA, H., YU, K.-P., MURPHY, M. LOIS, KARNOFSKY, D.: Daunomycin, an antitumour antibiotic in the treatment of neoplastic disease; clinical evaluation with special reference to childhood leukaemia. Cancer 20, 333 (1967).

TANAKA, N., YAMAGUCHI, H., UMEZAWA, H.: Mechanism of action of phleomycin, a tumour-inhibitory antibiotic. Biochem. Biophys. Res. Commun. 10, 171 (1963).

TARBELL, D. S., HOFFMAN, P., AL-KAZIMI, H. R., LEPAGE, G. A., ROSS, J. M., VOGT, H. R., WARGOTZ, B.: The chemistry of fumagillin. III. J. Amer. Chem. Soc. 77, 5610 (1955).

TARRO, G.: Effect of streptovitacin A on replication of an RNA virus (poliovirus). Proc. Soc. exp. Biol. (N. Y.) 126, 535 (1967).

TATSUOKA, S., NAKAZAWA, K., MIYAKE, A., KAZIWARA, K., ARAMAKI, Y., SHIBATA, M. TANABE, K., HAMADA, Y., HITOMI, H., MIYAMOTO, M., NIZUNO, K., WATANABE, J., ISHIDATE, M., YOKOTANI, H., ISHIKAWA, I.: Isolation, anticancer activity and pharmacology of a new antibiotic chromomycin. Gann 49, Suppl. 23 (1958).

TELLER, M. N.: Antibiotics in experimental cancer chemotherapy. Trans. N. Y. Acad. Sci. (2) 24, 158 (1961).

—, WAGSGUL, S. F., WOOLLEY, G. W.: Transplantable human tumours in experimental chemotherapy: effects of streptonigrin on HS/1 and HEp/3 in the rat. Antibiot. Chemother. 11, 165 (1961).

TENDLER, M. D., KORMAN, S.: Refuin: a noncytotoxic compound proliferated by a thermophilic actinomycete. Nature (Lond.) 199, 501 (1963).

THIELE, ELIZABETH H., ARISON, R. N., BOXER, G. E.: Oncolysis by Clostridia. III. Effects of Clostridia and chemotherapeutic agents on rodent tumours. Cancer Res. 24, 222 (1964 a).

— — — Oncolysis by Clostridia. IV. Effects of nonpathogenic clostridial spores in normal and pathological tissues. Cancer Res. 24, 234 (1964 b).

TODARO, G. J., BARON, S.: The role of interferon in the inhibition of SV40 transformation of mouse cell line 3T3. Proc. nat. Acad. Sci. (U. S.) 54, 752 (1965).

TOMKINS, G. M., MAXWELL, E. S.: Some aspects of steroid hormone action. Ann. Rev. Biochem. 32, 677 (1963).

TOYOSHIMA, S., SETO, Y., SAITO, K.: Antiviral effect of noformycin. Effective against both DNA and RNA viruses. Chemotherapy (Tokyo) 14, 457. Excerp. Med. 1967, Abst. 5140 (1966).

TRENTIN, J. J., YABE, Y., TAYLOR, G.: The quest for human cancer viruses. Science 137, 835 (1962).

TSUJIGUCHI, T.: Experimental studies on the resistance of tumour cells to anticancer drugs. Pt. I. Experimental studies on mitomycin C resistance of Yoshida sarcoma. Nagoya Igakkai Zasshi 83, 466 (1960); Cancer Chemotherapy Abstr. 2, 480 (1961).

TSUNODA, A.: Chemoprophylaxis of poliomyelitis in mice with quinomycin (Studies on the antibiotic from actinomyces). J. Antibiot. (Tokyo) A 15, 60 (1962).

TULINSKY, A.: The structure of mitomycin A. J. Amer. Chem. Soc. 84, 3188 (1962).

TYRRELL, D. A. J.: Interferon produced by cultures of calf kidney cells. Nature (Lond.) 184, 452 (1959).

—, WALKER, G. H., LEACH, B. E.: Efficacy of "Viractin" in preventing respiratory disease. Nature (Lond.) 210, 386 (1966).

UMEZAWA, H.: Bleomycin and other antitumour antibiotics of high molecular weight. In: Antimicrobial Agents and Chemotherapy, 1966, pp. 1079.

VAITKEVICIUS, V. K., REED, M. L.: Clinical studies with podophyllum compounds SP1-77 (NSC-72274) and SPG-827 (NSC-42076). Cancer Chemother. Rep. 50, 565 (1966).

VAN ROSSUM, W., DE SOMER, P.: Some aspects of the interferon production in vivo. Life Sci. 5, 105 (1966).

VARGA, A., HENRIKSEN, E.: Histologic observations on the effect of 17-α-hydroxyprogesterone-17-n-caproate on endometrial carcinoma. Obstet. Gynecol. 26, 656 (1965).

VENDITTI, J. M., GOLDIN, A.: Drug synergism in antineoplastic chemotherapy. Advanc. Chemotherapy 1, 397 (1964).

VESTER, F., NIENHAUS, J.: Cancerostatische Proteinkomponenten aus Viscum album. Experientia 21, 197 (1965).

VILCEK, J., FREER, J. H.: Inhibition of Sindbis virus plaque formation by extracts of E. coli. J. Bact. 92, 1716 (1966).

VILCEK, J., NG, M. H.: Potentiation of action of interferon by extracts of Escherichia coli. Virology 31, 552 (1967).

VOGEL, A. W.: Comparison of simultaneously incurred damage to bone marrow and tumour tissue of animals treated with anticancer agents. Cancer Res. 21, 636 (1961 a).

— Tumour-marrow index: a means of laboratory evaluation of antineoplastic compounds. Cancer Res. 21, 1450 (1961 b).

VON SALTZA, M. H., DUTCHER, P. D., REID, J.: The aminoheptose moiety of septacidin. Abst. 148th Amer. Chem. Soc. Meeting, Chicago, 15 Q (1964).

WADE, H. E., ELSWORTH, R., HERBERT, D., KEPPIE, J., SARGEANT, K.: A new L-asparaginase with antitumour activity. Lancet 2, 776 (1968).

WADE, R.: Hormones. In: Experimental Chemotherapy. Vol. V. Eds.: R. J. SCHNITZER and F. HAWKING. New York: Academic Press 1967, pp. 133—331.

WAGNER, R. R.: Inhibition of interferon biosynthesis by actinomycin D. Nature (Lond.) 204, 49 (1964).

—, LEVY, A. H., SNYDER, RUTH M., RATCLIFF, G. A., HYATT, D. F.: Biologic properties of two plaque variants of vesicular stomatitis virus (Indiana serotype). J. Immunol. 91, 112 (1963).

—, SNYDER, RUTH M., HOOK, E. W., LUTTRELL, C. N.: Effect of bacterial endotoxin in resistance of mice to viral encephalitides, including comparative studies of the interference phenomenon. J. Immunol. 83, 87 (1959).

WAKAHI, S., MARUMO, H., TOMIOKA, K., SHIMIZU, G., KATO, E., KAMADA, H., KUDO, S., FUJIMOTO, Y.: Isolation of new fractions of antitumour mitomycins. Antibiot. Chemother. 8, 228 (1958).

WAKISAKA, G., UCHINO, H., NAKAMURA, T., SOTOBAYASHI, H., SHIRAKAWA, S., ADACHI, A., SAKURAI, M.: Selective inhibition of biosynthesis of ribonucleic acid in mammalian cells by chromomycin A3. Nature (Lond.) 198, 385 (1963).

WAKSMAN, S. A., WOODRUFF, H. B.: Bacteriostatic and bactericidal substances produced by a soil actinomyces. Proc. Soc. exp. Biol. (N. Y.) 45, 609 (1940).

WALLER, C. W., FRYTH, P. W., HUTCHINGS, B. L., WILLIAMS, J. H.: Achromycin. The structure of the antibiotic puromycin. I. J. Amer. Chem. Soc. 75, 2025 (1953).

WARD, D. C., REICH, E., GOLDBERG, I. H.: Base specificity in the interaction of polynucleotides with antibiotic drugs. Science 149, 1259 (1965).

WATNE, A. L., MOORE, D., GORGUN, B.: Solid tumour chemotherapy with mitomycin C. Arch. Surg. 95, 175 (1967).

WATSON, G. F.: Preliminary report on the effect of concentrated calf spleen extract on spontaneous mouse tumours. Growth 30, 491 (1966).

WEBB, A. E., WETHERLEY-MEIN, G., GORDON-SMITH, C. E., MCMAHON, D.: Leukaemia and neoplastic processes treated with Langat and Kyasanur forest disease viruses. A clinical and laboratory study of 28 patients. Brit. med. J. 1, 258 (1966).

WEBB, J. L.: Enzyme and metabolic inhibitors, Vol. 1. New York: Academic Press 1963, pp. 498—500.

WEBB, J. S., COSULICH, D. B., MOWAT, J. H., PATRICK, J. B., BROSCHARD, R. W., MEYER, W. E., WILLIAMS, R. P., WOLF, C. F., FULMOR, W., PIDACKS, C., LANCASTER, J. E.: The structure of mitomycins A, B, C and Porfiromycin. Pts. I and II. J. Amer. Chem. Soc. 84, 3185, 3187 (1962).

WECKER, E.: Effect of puromycin on the replication of Western equine encephalitis and poliomyelitis viruses. Nature (Lond.) 197, 1277 (1963).

WEHRLI, W., NÜESCH, J., KNÜSEL, F.: Action of rifampicin on RNA polymerase. Biochem. biophys. Acta 157, 215 (1968).

WEISSBACH, A., LISIO, A.: Alkylation of nucleic acids by mitomycin C and porfiromycin. Biochemistry 4, 196 (1965).

WERNER, G. H., GANTER, P., DE RATULD, Y.: Studies on the antiviral activity of distamycin A. Chemotherapia 9, 65 (1964).

WHEELOCK, E. F.: Effect of statolon on Friend virus leukaemia in mice. Proc. Soc. exp. Biol. (N. Y.) 124, 855 (1967).

WHITE, F. R.: Actinomycin D. Cancer Chemother. Rep. 5, 53 (1959 a).

— Mitomycin C. Cancer Chemother. Rep. 2, 21 (1959 b).

— Actidione. Cancer Chemother. Rep. 5, 59 (1959 c).

WILLIAMS, H. M.: Combination vinblastine-chlorambucil therapy in solid tumours. Proc. Amer. Ass. Cancer Res. 5, 68 (1964).

WILLIAMS-ASHMAN, H. G.: New facets of the biochemistry of steroid hormone action. Cancer Res. 25, 1096 (1965).

WILSON, H. E., LOUIS, J.: The response of Hodgkin's disease to treatment with oral vinblastine sulphate. Ann. int. Med. 67, 303 (1967).

WILSON, W. L., LABRA, C., BARRIST, E.: Preliminary observations on the use of streptonigrin as an antitumour agent in human beings. Antibiot. Chemother. 11, 147 (1961).

WOLSTENHOLME, G. E. W., O'CONNOR, MAEVE (Eds.): Interferon. Ciba Foundation Symposium. London: Churchill 1968.

WOOD, S. J., JR.: Pathogenesis of metastasis formation observed in vivo in the rabbit ear-chamber. Arch. Path. (Chicago) 66, 550 (1958).

WOODRUFF, M. F. A., BOAK, J. L.: Inhibitory effect of injection of Corynebacterium parvum on the growth of tumour transplants in isogenic hosts. Brit. J. Cancer 20, 345 (1966).

YAMAMOTO, H., MATSUMAE, A., HATA, T.: Cephalomycin, an antiviral antibiotic. III. Further purification of cephalomycin. J. Antibiot. (Tokyo) A 16, 121 (1963).

YAMAZAKI, S., NITTA, K., HIKIJI, T., NOGI, M., TAKEUCHI, T., YAMAZAKI, S., NITTA, K., HIKIJI, T., NOGI, M., TAKEUCHI, T., YAMAMOTO, T., UMEZAWA, H.: Cylinder plate method of testing the anti-cell effect. Studies on antitumour substances produced by Actinomycetes. XII. J. Antibiot. (Tokyo) A 9, 135 (1956).

YANO, M., KUSAKIRI, T., MIURA, Y.: Intracellular transfer of nucleic acids in rat ascites hepatoma cells. J. Biochem. 53, 461 (1963).

YARBRO, J. W., KENNEDY, B. J., BARNUM, C. P.: Mithramycin: inhibitor of ribonucleic acid synthesis. Cancer Res. 26, 36 (1966).

YARDEN, A., LAVIE, D.: Constituents of Withania sonnifera. Pt. I. The functional groups of withaferin. J. Chem. Soc., Pt. III, 2925 (1962).

YARNELL, M., AMBROSE, E. J., SHEPLEY, K., TACHO, R.: Drug assays on organ cultures of biopsies from human tumours. Brit. med. J. 2, 490 (1964).

YELLIN, T. O., WRISTON, J. C.: Antagonism of purified asparaginase from guinea-pig serum towards lymphoma. Science 151, 998 (1966).

YOUNGNER, J. S., HALLUM, J. V.: Interferon production in mice by double-stranded synthetic polynuclectides: induction or release? Virology 35, 177 (1968).

—, STINEBRING, W. R.: Interferon production in chickens infected with Brucella abortus. Science 144, 1022 (1964).

— —, TAUBE, SHEILA E.: Influence of inhibitors of protein synthesis on interferon formation in mice. Virology 27, 541 (1965).

YOUNT, W. J., FINKEL, H. E.: Treatment of refractory reticulum cell sarcoma with low doses of vincristine sulphate. J. Amer. med. Ass. 197, 535 (1966).

ZAKAY-RONESS, Z., BERNKOPF, H.: Effect of active and ultraviolet irradiated inactive vaccinia virus on the development of Shay leukaemia in rats. Cancer Res. 24, 373 (1964).

ZAMECNIK, P. C.: Unsettled questions in the field of protein synthesis. The first Jubilee lecture. Biochem. J. 85, 257 (1962).

ZISCHKA, ROSEMARIE, LANGLOIS, A. J., RAO, P. R., BONAR, R. A., BEARD, J. W.: Effects of actinomycin D on avian myeloblast and BAI strain A virus RNA synthesis in vitro. Cancer Res. 26, 1839 (1966).

Subject Index

Type-setting: Konrad Triltsch, Graphischer Betrieb, 87 Würzburg, Germany

Monographs already Published

1 SCHINDLER, R., Lausanne: Die tierische Zelle in Zellkultur. DM 16,—; US $ 4.40

2 Neuroblastomas — Biochemical Studies. Edited by C. BOHUON, Villejuif (Symposium). DM 16,—; US $ 4.40

3 HUEPER, W. C., Bethesda: Occupational and Environmental Cancers of the Respiratory System. DM 34,—; US $ 9.40

4 GOLDMAN, L., Cincinnati: Laser Cancer Research. DM 16,—; US $ 5.00

5 METCALF, D., Melbourne: The Thymus. Its Role in Immune Responses, Leukaemia Development and Carcinogenesis. DM 24,—; US $ 6.60

6 Malignant Transformation by Viruses. Edited by W. H. KIRSTEN, Chicago (Symposium). DM 32,—; US $ 8.80

7 MOERTEL, CH. G., Rochester: Multiple Primary Malignant Neoplasms. Their Incidence and Significance. DM 18,—; US $ 5.00

8 New Trends in the Treatment of Cancer. Edited by L. MANUILA, S. MOLES, and P. RENTCHNICK, Geneva. DM 32,—; US $ 8.80

9 LINDENMANN, J., Zürich, and P. A. KLEIN, Gainesville/Florida: Immunological Aspects of Viral Oncolysis. DM 18,—; US $ 5.00

10 NELSON, R. S., Houston: Radioactive Phosphorus in the Diagnosis of Gastrointestinal Cancer. DM 15,—; US $ 4.20

11 FREEMAN, R. G., and J. M. KNOX, Houston: Treatment of Skin Cancer. DM 15,—; US $ 4.50

12 LYNCH, H. T., Houston: Hereditary Factors in Carcinoma. DM 24,—; US $ 6.60

13 Tumours in Children. Edited by H. B. MARSDEN, and J. K. STEWARD, Manchester. DM 72,—; US $ 18.00

14 ODARTCHENKO, N., Lausanne: Production cellulaire érythropoïétique. DM 28,—; US $ 7.70

15 SOKOLOFF, B., Lakeland/Florida: Carcinoid and Serotonin. DM 24,—; US $ 6.60

16 JACOBS, M. L., Duarte/California: Malignant Lymphomas and their Management. DM 18,—; US $ 5.10

17 Normal and Malignant Cell Growth. Edited by R. J. M. FRY, Argonne, M. L. GRIEM, Argonne, and W. H. KIRSTEN, Chicago (Symposium). DM 56,80; US $ 14.20

18 ANGLESIO, E., Torino: The Treatment of Hodgkin's Disease. DM 24,—; US $ 6.60

19 BANNASCH, P., Würzburg: The Cytoplasm of Hepatocytes during Carcinogenesis. DM 32,—; US $ 8.80

20 Rubidomycin. A new Agent against Leukemia. Edited by J. BERNARD, R. PAUL, M. BOIRON, C. JACQUILLAT, and R. MARAL, Paris. DM 48,—; US $ 13.20

21 Scientific Basis of Cancer Chemotherapy. Edited by G. MATHÉ, Villejuif (Symposium). DM 28,—; US $ 7.00

22 KOLDOVSKÝ, P., Philadelphia: Tumor Specific Transplantation Antigen. DM 24,—; US $ 6.60

23 FUCHS, W. A., Bern, J. W. DAVIDSON, Toronto, and H. W. FISCHER, Ann Arbor: Lymphography in Cancer. DM 76,—; US $ 21.00

25 ROY-BURMAN, P., Los Angeles: Analogues of Nucleic Acid Components. Mechanisms of Action. DM 28,—; US $ 7.70

26 Tumors of the Liver. Edited by G. T. PACK and A. H. ISLAMI, New York.
DM 56,—; US $ 15.40

28 MEEK, E. S., Bristol: Antitumour and Antiviral Substances of Natural Origin.
DM 16,—; US $ 4.40

In Production

24 HAYWARD, J. L., London: Hormonal Research in Human Breast Cancer

27 SZYMENDERA, J., Warsaw: Bone Mineral Metabolism in Cancer. DM 32,—;
US $ 8.80

29 Aseptic Environments and Cancer Treatment. Edited by G. MATHÉ, Villejuif
(Symposium)

30 Advances in the Treatment of Acute (Blastic) Leukaemias. Edited by G. MATHÉ,
Villejuif (Symposium)

31 DENOIX, P., Villejuif: Treatment of Malignant Breast Tumors: Indications and
Results

In Preparation

ACKERMANN, N. B., Boston: Use of Radioisotopic Agents in the Diagnosis of
Cancer

Asparaginase. Edited by E. GRUNDMANN, Wuppertal-Elberfeld, and H. F.
OETTGEN, New York (Symposium)

BOIRON, M., Paris: The Viruses of the Leukemia-sarcoma Complex

CAVALIERE, R., A. ROSSI-FANELLI, B. MONDOVI, and G. MORICCA, Roma: Selective Heat Sensitivity of Cancer Cells

CHIAPPA, S., Milano: Endolymphatic Radiotherapy in Malignant Lymphomas

Cutane paraneoplastische Syndrome. Edited by J. J. HERZBERG. Bremen (Symposium)

GRUNDMANN, E., Wuppertal-Elberfeld: Morphologie und Cytochemie der Car-
cinogenese

IRLIN, I. S., Moskva: Mechanisms of Viral Carcinogenesis

LANGLEY, F. A., and A. C. CROMPTON, Manchester: Epithelial Abnormalities
of the Cervix Uteri

MATHÉ, G., Villejuif: L'Immunothérapie des Cancers

NELSON, R. S., Houston: Endoscopy in Gastric Cancer

NEWMAN, M. K., Detroit: Neuropathies and Myopathies Associated with
Occult Malignancies

OGAWA, K., Osaka: Ultrastructural Enzyme Cytochemistry of Azo-dye Carcinogenesis

PENN, I., Denver: Malignant Lymphomas in Transplant Patients

Recent Advances in the Treatment of Acute Leukemias. Edited by G. MATHÉ,
Villejuif (Symposium)

SUGIMURA, T., Tokyo, H. ENDO, Fukuoka, and T. ONO, Tokyo: Chemistry and
Biological Action of 4-Nitroquinoline 1-oxide, a Carcinogen

WEIL, R., Lausanne: Biological and Structural Properties of Polyoma Virus and
its DNA

WILLIAMS, D. C., Caterham, Surrey: The Basis for Therapy of Hormon Sensitive Tumours

WILLIAMS, D. C., Caterham, Surrey: The Biochemistry of Metastasis

GPSR Compliance
The European Union's (EU) General Product Safety Regulation (GPSR) is a set
of rules that requires consumer products to be safe and our obligations to
ensure this.

If you have any concerns about our products, you can contact us on

ProductSafety@springernature.com

In case Publisher is established outside the EU, the EU authorized
representative is:

Springer Nature Customer Service Center GmbH
Europaplatz 3
69115 Heidelberg, Germany